Jane

MEASURING PATIENT OUTCOMES

MEASURING PATIENT OUTCOMES

Marie T. Nolan • Victoria Mock

Sage Publications, Inc.
International Educational and Professional Publisher
Thousand Oaks ■ London ■ New Delhi

For information:

Sage Publications, Inc.
2455 Teller Road
Thousand Oaks, California 91320
E-mail: order@sagepub.com

Sage Publications Ltd.
6 Bonhill Street
London EC2A 4PU
United Kingdom

Sage Publications India Pvt. Ltd.
M-32 Market
Greater Kailash I
New Delhi 110 048 India

Printed in the United States of America

Library of Congress Cataloging-in-Publication Data

Main entry under title:
    Measuring patient outcomes / [edited] by Marie T. Nolan
and Victoria Mock.
        p.   cm.
    Includes bibliographical references and index.
    ISBN 0-7619-1505-2 (pbk.: acid-free paper)
    1. Outcome assessment (Medical care) I. Nolan, Marie T.
II. Mock, Victoria. III. Title
R853.O87 M43   2000
362.1—dc21   99-006844

This book is printed on acid-free paper.

00   01   02   03   04   05   06   7   6   5   4   3   2   1

Acquiring Editor: C. Deborah Laughton
Editorial Assistant: Eileen Carr
Production Editor: Astrid Virding
Editorial Assistant: Cindy Bear
Typesetter: Lynn Miyata
Cover Designer: Michelle Lee

To my husband, Patrick G. Nolan,
and to my parents,
Alice M. Gould, RN, BA, and James P. Gould, MD,
my first and best example of the multidisciplinary team.

—Marie T. Nolan

To my husband, Quent, and my son, Grey,
for their loving support and the joy they bring to my life.

—Victoria Mock

Finally, to the clinical nurses and graduate students
who vigilantly measure patient outcomes
to continually improve the care of their patients.

Contents

PART II: CASE STUDIES IN PATIENT OUTCOMES MANAGEMENT   103

Acute Care

Maternal and Child Care

Primary Care

Foreword

It is a privilege to introduce a book that deals with the practical issues and basic tools of measuring patient outcomes. This book is a clear, step-by-step primer to organize the reader's thinking about kinds of outcome assessment, the nature and scope of measurement, and the context and processes of interdisciplinary care—all necessary components to understand before engaging in the tasks entailed in patient outcomes research. The clinical examples operationalize the how-to's into real-life patient care situations. To advance practice nurses everywhere: This is the book you have been waiting for! It is the guide for measuring patient outcomes as we enter the 21st century.

Throughout the 1980s and the 1990s, advance practice nurses (APNs) and nurse researchers employed in clinical settings struggled to appropriately identify, elicit, aggregate, and illustrate data from existing clinical sources to present the most accurate depiction of patient care outcomes. Often, they were faced with clinical data that did not translate across patient populations, that were incomplete or missing, and that were suspect as to their conceptual clarity when viewed within the context of diagnostic groups, gender, or age.

Two challenges were paramount for the pioneers of patient outcomes research. The first challenge was to understand fully, embrace, and integrate the concept of measurement into the clinical arena. This meant moving the clinical environment beyond the proliferation of unreliable and invalid questionnaires to one of devising or selecting reliable, valid, and practical tools for use with patients. The second challenge was to understand fully, embrace, and integrate the concept of cost into the practice environment. This meant transforming from holding negative ideas about cost-related decisions into learning how to collect, analyze, and relate cost data to practice and care outcome variables. During the 1980s and 1990s, we evolved from an opinion-related process of writing letters to influence decisions for or against an impending architectural or practice change that affected the care we gave to our patients to a data-driven process of explicitly and systematically collecting data to influence decisions.

As I read this book, I was reminded of the influences of the previous decades that have led us to measure patient outcomes in the 21st century. The atmosphere of the 1980s was one focused on the integration of research in practice, including partnerships of APNs and academicians, with a huge influx of doctorally prepared nurses hired into clinical settings to lead this integration. While the scientific community sent out a plea for the development of reliable and valid tools to measure abstract care concepts, desperately needed in clinical research, we celebrated the congressional approval of the National Center for Nursing Research (NCNR) at the National Institutes of Health (NIH). More than 100 APNs, administrators, educators, and nurse researchers were mentored in their development and testing of psychometrically sound instruments through the Measurement of Clinical and Educational Nursing Outcomes Project, administered by Drs. Carolyn Waltz and Ora Strickland at the University of Maryland, School of Nursing and funded by the Division of Nursing, Special Projects Branch. These tools now serve as a rich resource for today's studies of patient outcomes. Under the leadership of NCNR Director Dr. Ada Sue Hinshaw, NCNR led the way in examining a research agenda for outcomes research in the early 1990s. It was during this time that NCNR became an institute (NINR) within the NIH. NCNR invited collaboration with the Agency for Health Care Policy and Research, and together they sponsored the first national conference on patient outcomes research: Examining the Effectiveness of Nursing Practice. This NIH-supported conference brought together scholars from throughout the United States to discuss the seedlings of the fruit we bear today. The visibility and influence of nurse scholars as viable members of the interdisciplinary scientific health community in all these events set the stage for a collaborative effort in addressing the measurement of patient outcomes in the clinical arenas of the 21st century.

Doctors Marie Nolan and Victoria Mock have given us a wonderful gift to guide us into the 21st century. This book brings together the experience of health care professionals and the latest knowledge about what is necessary to

- Identify and measure patient outcomes successfully and practically

- Analyze and illustrate reliable and valid outcomes data using the latest technology and computer packages

- Use the results of systematic, interdisciplinary outcomes studies to improve care and plan future studies

Measuring Patient Outcomes delivers an enthusiastic message about the strength of interdisciplinary teams and the power of reliable and valid data to make decisions that affect the care outcomes of our patients. This is the message of patient outcomes research in the 21st Century!

—Veronica F. Rempusheski, *PhD, RN, FAAN*
Associate Professor
University of Rochester School of Nursing
Rochester, New York

Preface

In our roles as nurse researchers at The Johns Hopkins Hospital and faculty members at The Johns Hopkins University School of Nursing, we are commonly called on to assist case managers, clinical nurse specialists, nurse managers, and students in the measurement of patient outcomes. We noted that although there is a great deal of literature describing managed care systems, case management, and the role of the advance practice nurse and nurse manager in the coordination of care, there was little that explained how to measure outcomes in a practical sense. Over time, we created materials to guide nurses and other clinicians through this process. These materials included information on how to select outcomes to improve, how to find instruments to accurately measure these outcomes, and how to select the statistical procedures to analyze these outcomes. Because successful measurement of patient outcomes requires a minimal level of data competence, we also have taught clinicians and students how to use the statistical analysis computer program, SPSS®, to analyze patient outcomes data and create graphics to summarize these data. This book is a compilation of the materials that we have used to teach patient outcomes measurement with additional information to help the reader get started.

The first part of this book serves as a primer for nurses and other health professionals who are ready to begin measuring patient outcomes. The second part of the book includes a series of case studies describing successful patient outcomes projects. The examples we have selected range from the straightforward assessment of length of stay and readmission rate before and after the introduction of a care pathway to the more complicated efforts to assess the impact of swimming on central venous catheter infection in children with cancer. Some chapters represent the starting point for outcomes measurement. whereas other chapters are built on previous work. Because we are continually impressed with the resourcefulness of clinicians who overcome barriers to the measurement of outcomes, we have included projects that highlight their strategies for success. Although some project leaders accessed existing clinical databases, two project leaders were assisted by graduate students who conducted chart reviews and one project leader was assisted by a medical student who performed data entry. One project leader used an informational cancer web site to identify an outcome of importance to cancer patients. Another coordinated the efforts of health professionals across five settings to study factors that were related to leg wound complications following coronary artery bypass graft. We know readers will benefit from these examples of outcomes measurement, and we wish our readers much success in their own outcomes measurement achievements.

About the Authors

Marie T. Nolan, DNSc, is Assistant Professor at The Johns Hopkins University School of Nursing and Nurse Researcher for Nursing Administration at The Johns Hopkins Hospital. Her research focuses on patient outcomes in serious illness. She has studied the stress experienced by patients and their families awaiting heart transplantation and patient decision making in patients with terminal illness. She teaches graduate courses in patient outcomes measurement and case management. She is coeditor (with Sharon M. Augustine) of *Transplantation Nursing: Acute and Long-Term Management* (1995). Her recent work has been published in the *Journal of Professional Nursing, Nursing Outlook, Nursing Economics, Dimensions of Critical Care, Heart & Lung,* and *Academic Medicine.*

Victoria Mock, DNSc, RN, AOCN, is Associate Director at The Johns Hopkins University School of Nursing, and at the School of Medicine. She is also Director of Nursing Research at the Johns Hopkins Comprehensive Cancer Center. She was appointed an American Cancer Society Professor of Oncology Nursing in 1999. Her research focuses on symptom management and quality of life. She is principal investigator of a multi-institutional clinical trial investigating the effects of exercise on fatigue and other symptoms during cancer treatment. She is also coinvestigator of another multisite study—the Oncology Nursing Society (ONS) Acute Care/Radiation Therapy Outcomes Research Project. She received the 1997 ONS Schering Excellence in Cancer Nursing Research Award and the 1998 ONS Ortho Biotech FIRE (Fatigue Initiative in Research and Education) Cancer Excellence Award. Her work appears in numerous books and journals.

List of Case Study Authors

Donna L. Brannan, RN, MSN
Nursing Staff Assistant
Neurosciences and Psychiatry Nursing
The Johns Hopkins Hospital
Baltimore, MD

Laura J. Burke, RN, PhD, FAAN
Director of Nursing Research
Aurora Health Care—Metro Region
West Allis, WI

Susan M. Cohen, DSN, RN
Associate Professor
Director, Adult and Family Nurse Practitioner Program
School of Nursing
Yale University
New Haven, CT

JoAnn Coleman, RN, MS, ACNP-CS, AOCN
Acute Care Nurse Practitioner, Pancreas and Biliary Surgery
Department of Surgical Nursing
The Johns Hopkins Hospital
Baltimore, MD

Philene Cromwell, MS, RN
Advanced Practice Nurse
Associate Clinical Professor
University of Rochester School of Nursing
University of Rochester Medical Center
Division of Pediatric Hematology/Oncology
Rochester, NY

Christine A. Engstrom, RN, MS, CRNP, AOCN
Adult Nurse Practitioner
Department of Medical Oncology
Baltimore Veterans Administration Medical Center
Baltimore, MD

Maura Goldsborough, RN, MSN
Research Nurse Program Coordinator
Cardiac Surgery
The Johns Hopkins Hospital
Baltimore, MD

Andrea O. Hollingsworth, PhD, RN
Associate Professor
Director, Undergraduate Nursing Program
College of Nursing
Villanova University
Villanova, PA

Marinell H. Jernigan, RN, EdD
Thesis Chair
University of North Carolina at Charlotte
Charlotte, NC

David N. Korones, MD
Assistant Professor of Pediatrics
University of Rochester School of Medicine and Dentistry
University of Rochester Medical Center
Division of Pediatric Hematology/Oncology
Rochester, NY

Penny Marschke, RN, MSN
Clinical Research Program Coordinator
Department of Urology
The Johns Hopkins University School of Medicine
Doctoral Candidate in Nursing
University of Maryland
Baltimore, MD

Barbara F. Paegelow, A.R.T.
Clinical Data Specialist
Aurora Health Care - Metro Region
Milwaukee, WI

Jacqueline Robbins, MS, RN CPNP
Pediatric Nurse Practitioner
Associate Clinical Professor
University of Rochester School of Nursing
University of Rochester Medical Center
Division of Pediatric Hematology/Oncology
Rochester, NY

Judith M. Rohde, RN, MSN
Director of Nursing
Neuroscience and Psychiatry Nursing
The Johns Hopkins Hospital
Baltimore, MD

Pamela T. Rudisill, RN, MSN, CCRN, ANP
Associate Executive Director of Nursing
Lake Norman Regional Medical Center
Mooresville, NC

Suzanne J. Rumble, RN, MSN, CCRN
Nursing Instructor
Presbyterian Hospital School of Nursing
Charlotte, NC

PART I

The Process of Patient Outcomes Management

CHAPTER 1

The Identification
of Patient Outcomes

Marie T. Nolan
Victoria Mock

The presentation of patient outcomes data can be tremendously empowering to those with an appreciation for its impact. Like the colors on the artist's palette, data can be used to create a picture that will inspire, persuade, inflame, or call the viewer to action. This does not mean that data can be manipulated to indicate whatever one chooses. Rather, like the completed painting, when presented well, data invite the viewer to participate in interpretation. For multidisciplinary groups, interpretation of patient outcomes data is a starting point in the improvement of patient care. For example, viewing the data on length of stay for patients in a particular diagnostic-related group (DRG) can stimulate a lively discussion of factors that influence length of stay, such as age, chronic illness, social support, and acute care interventions.

Nurses have long been concerned with patient responses to treatment and illness, but they have infrequently been positioned to make systemwide changes to influence these outcomes. The ability to analyze and present data is a creative skill that brings both nurse clinicians and executives to the fore in the move to improve patient outcomes. Several case managers and clinical nurse specialists have reported that nurse executives, physicians, and hospital administrators began to view them as leaders in the organization when they began presenting patient outcomes data at meetings and in reports. Similarly, executives in nursing have found that analysis and dissemination of patient outcomes data to key decision makers is increasingly important when building support for new programs (Erickson, 1998).

In a recent consultation from the director of case management of a neighboring hospital, the director requested assistance in increasing her program's impact on patient outcomes. Her staff included several specialty-based case managers who, during the past 2 years, had worked on the multidisciplinary development and implementation of several critical pathways. The director believed that the case managers had successfully rooted out much inefficiency in patient care processes. She had little data to support this contention, however. Our recommendations to the director were that by developing skills in the art of managing, analyzing, and presenting patient outcomes data, she and the case managers could more effectively lead multidisciplinary groups working to improve outcomes. Having this type of data in hand would enable the director to evaluate and expand the boundaries of the overall case management program to allow for greater impact on patient care throughout the organization.

BACKGROUND

During the early years of managed care there was a flurry of activity focused on containing rapidly increasing health care costs. Although health care organizations increased their efficiency and integrated services to streamline care and improve outcomes, it was the draconian measures employed by some managed care organizations that made headlines in the daily news. Reports of patients who were denied needed care and of managed care contracts with gag rules preventing physicians from recommending care that was not covered by a patient's health plan seriously eroded the trust that patients had traditionally placed in health professionals and health care institutions (Moran, 1998).

In the aftermath of this era of tightly controlled access to care, we are beginning to see new types of health care networks emerging. For example, less restrictive preferred provider organizations (PPOs) now have 40% more members than health maintenance organizations (HMOs) (Freudenheim, 1998). A gatekeeper physician does not control the care of PPO members, and, for a fee, members can seek care from doctors and hospitals outside the network. This new era of choice means that measuring the quality of care is now more important than ever. Employers remain interested in holding down the cost of health care for employees, and patients will choose the providers who can assist them in obtaining the best health care. If we are to reclaim the public's trust, the new charge for health care organizations is to manage costs in a manner that is fiscally responsible while demonstrating positive patient outcomes.

As clinical nurse researchers, the direction we have provided to individual case managers, clinical specialists, nurse executives, and others led to the development of this book to guide those charged with measuring and managing patient outcomes in their organization. The structure of any patient outcomes management program should address the following key issues, which are introduced in this chapter and explained further throughout the book:

- Types of outcomes identified
- Multidisciplinary approaches and benchmarking
- Outcomes management and outcomes research
- Ethical issues in the selection and use of patient outcomes

TYPES OF OUTCOMES IDENTIFIED

Outcomes are the end result of care, or a measurable change in the health status or behavior of patients (Harris, 1991). Mortality and morbidity are patient outcomes that have been traditionally used to examine the effect of medical interventions. Although these outcomes provide a gross measure of the quality of care delivered, they focus primarily on physiologic or clinical outcomes and do not describe how an illness or stressor has impacted other areas of the patient's life. Brooten and Naylor (1995) note that because mortality rates are generally low, large sample sizes in multi-institutional studies are required to demonstrate significant differences across institutions. Similarly, health services research employs large administrative databases to compare one type of plan with another (e.g., capitation vs. fee-for-service plans). These studies measure the impact of an overall plan but provide little information about how the specific elements of a plan influence patient outcomes (Pincus, Zarin, & West, 1996).

Hegyvary (1991) proposed four categories of outcome assessment that reflect the perspectives of the patient, the providers, and the purchasers of health care:

1. Clinical: the patient's response to medical and nursing interventions
2. Functional: the patient's maintenance or improvement of physical functioning
3. Financial: outcomes achieved with the most efficient use of resources
4. Perceptual: the patient's satisfaction with outcomes, care received, and providers

Examples of clinical outcomes are wound healing, mobility, weight gain, body temperature, blood pressure, heart rate, blood sugar, and peak expiratory flow rate. Functional outcomes can be specific, such as the ability to perform self-catheterization independently, or global, such as an overall sense of well-being and independent living skills at 1 year following heart transplantation. Financial outcomes include the direct costs of delivering care or outcomes that approximate cost of care, such as length of hospital stay or frequency of emergency department visits in a year.

Finally, perceptual outcomes gained new attention in the wake of public outcry regarding limitations on hospital stays following childbirth. The subsequent legislation guaranteeing 48-hour maternal inpatient care was a wake-up call for managed care organizations. In addressing the debate regarding "drive-through deliveries," health policy analyst Jan Greene (1997) explained,

> HMO leaders should have realized the issue wasn't about the medical necessity of 48-hour maternity stays. They should have recognized that the one time a woman actually wants to be in the hospital is when she is ready to give birth. (p. 40)

Member satisfaction is one of the key indicators of a managed care organization's quality as reviewed by the National Committee for Quality Assurance (NCQA), the private, not-for-profit organization that accredits managed care organizations.

Outcomes can immediately follow an intervention or occur long after an intervention has been performed. Pain level with the use of patient-controlled analgesia after surgery represents an immediate outcome, whereas functional status at 6 months following hip replacement represents a long-term outcome. Both the type and the timing of the outcomes to be measured influence how the outcome should be measured. The following are other questions that must be addressed before finalizing the selection of a patient outcome to be measured: Is there an existing instrument to measure this or will one have to be developed? Are there costs involved in measuring the outcome? For example, to assess the outcome of average daily peak inspiratory flow in children with asthma, a peak flowmeter will have to be purchased for each child. Also, will the measure be subjective or objective and who will perform the measurement, one person or many individuals? If many individuals will be measuring the outcome, some time may be needed to train those involved to ensure a reasonable degree of interrater reliability. If outcomes are to be measured across settings—for example, in the hospital and in the home—is there cooperation among the care providers in the various settings regarding the measurement? A multidisciplinary effort may be required for some outcomes projects.

MULTIDISCIPLINARY APPROACHES
AND BENCHMARKING

Multidisciplinary Groups

Multidisciplinary groups are a necessity when selecting and evaluating patient outcomes that are influenced by the practice of more than one health professional. Omitting key caregivers from the planning of outcomes evaluation can result in the omission of essential aspects of the outcome being studied. Several clinical chapters in this book reflect the work of multidisciplinary groups. The outcome of regaining continence following prostate surgery (Chapter 9, this volume), central-venous catheter infections in children with cancer (Chapter 11, this volume), and quality of life following surgery for pancreatic disease (Chapter 12, this volume) are just a few examples of outcomes that can be influenced through multidisciplinary approaches to care. An added benefit of careful multidisciplinary planning at the outset is the pooling of resources to measure the outcomes of interest. Several of the clinical chapters describe creative ways to complete tasks such as data entry and analysis.

Nurses are in the ideal position to lead multidisciplinary groups in measuring and managing patient outcomes. Jennings (1991) noted that, "Nurses have a solid sense of the illness trajectory, because it is primarily nursing care that is delivered in community settings and the home" (p. 70). For example, working closely with oncology medical specialists, oncology nurse outcomes managers influence patient comfort, length of stay, and cost of care. They help identify effective drug therapy for symptom management in patients, and they provide comprehensive patient education to enable patients to cope with their cancer. These interventions result in reduced hospital admissions and improved health status (Lasker-Hertz & Houston, 1995).

Benchmarking Against the Outcomes of Other Organizations

Multidisciplinary groups can be extended to multi-institutional groups. Benchmarking involves comparing an organization's patient outcomes against those of a similar organization or against those of an organization that is known as a center of excellence in a particular area of patient care. This can be used as a means of identifying an organization's areas of weakness and prioritizing patient outcomes on which to focus. For example, in 1992 several children's hospitals throughout the country formed a cooperative group to share data concerning the quality of care in their institutions. The outcomes they have examined include nosocomial infections, parent and patient satisfaction, unplanned returns, and costs of care (Porter, 1995). When one of the children's hospitals is identified as being a "best practice" institution in one of these areas, key clinical and managerial staff of that institution are assembled to share information about processes with the other member hospitals. Using a slightly different strategy, three hospitals in Syracuse, New York, banded together to compare their care and outcomes data with similar data from three hospitals in California and Washington (Lagoe & Aspling, 1997). Two of the comparison hospitals were chosen because they had similar patient populations. The third comparison hospital in San Diego, California, was chosen because it had one of the shortest acute care stays in the nation. The hospitals examined medical and surgical patients within DRGs representing high volumes of patients in their facilities, such as pneumonia, myocardial infarction, and hip replacement. The authors reported that benchmarking was useful in reducing surgical costs but not medical costs. They attributed this result to the fact that medical patients have more comorbidities and are often nonelective admissions for whom care is difficult to predict.

Patient outcomes data that can be used for making comparisons are also available on the Internet. The Agency for Health Care Policy and Research (1998) provides on-line data describing the mean length of stay and the mean charges by DRG. The advantage of this site is that it represents very large data sets. One sample included more than 34 million patients. A disadvantage, however, is the age of the data. No posted data set was less than 4 years old. Another on-line site for outcomes data is provided by the NCQA, the accrediting body for managed care organizations. NCQA maintains a database of 71 performance indicators for managed care organizations, such as member satisfaction and frequency of childhood immunizations and cesarean sections. A sample of the data on-line is provided free of charge. More extensive information is available to members for a fee, however.

OUTCOMES MANAGEMENT AND OUTCOMES RESEARCH

There is much in common between outcomes management and outcomes research. Both can involve research methods and the evaluation of similar patient outcomes. Some researchers have distinguished the two, based on the extent of the scientific rigor used in the exploration of outcomes (Erickson, 1998). Others have emphasized the interdependence of the two approaches (Lasker-Hertz & Houston, 1995). In some instances, outcomes management can be the starting point for outcomes research simply by identifying problems or issues in need of more in-depth exploration. For example, an outcomes project might reveal that patients hospitalized with myocardial infarction who have concurrent chronic obstructive pulmonary disease (COPD) are re-admitted within 30 days of hospitalization more frequently than are patients without COPD. This finding suggests the need for a research project to more precisely study the impact of COPD on recovery after myocardial infarction. In other instances, outcomes research can serve as the starting point for outcomes management. For example, studies of a particular treatment's efficacy provide the essential foundation for studies of the treatment's effectiveness.

Efficacy Versus Effectiveness Studies

Efficacy studies are generally carried out by researchers who treat selected patients who are randomly assigned to receive an experimental treatment according to strict protocols. In contrast, effectiveness studies view treatments as they are provided in usual practice settings (Epstein & Sherwood, 1996). Many studies of patient outcomes that are led by outcomes managers are evaluations of effectiveness. These studies provide important information about patient perceptions of and compliance with a particular treatment. Also, treatment barriers in the practice setting can be identified and potentially modified to maximize the impact of the intervention.

The Need for Institutional Review Board Approval

As nurse researchers, we are frequently asked to decide whether a proposal for an outcomes study should be sent to the institutional review board (IRB) for approval. Although there is little published information on this specific question, issues to be addressed include

- The nature of the treatment used, if any (standard vs. experimental)
- The patient burden and risks involved
- The protection of patient identity

If a treatment or intervention is used that is considered experimental or not consistent with the current standard of care, the proposal should be submitted to the IRB. Also, if the patient burden involved is significant, the proposal should be submitted to the IRB. An example of an outcomes study with a patient burden that is not significant is one in which patients complete a satisfaction survey upon or shortly after discharge from a hospital. In contrast, an example of an outcomes study with a patient burden that is significant is one in which patients complete several surveys or in which repeated measures are necessary, such as ongoing symptom evaluation in patients who fatigue easily.

Any outcomes study that has the potential of revealing the patient's identity should be reviewed by the IRB. An example of this type is a study of functional status outcomes following rare treatments such as heart transplantation. In publications of this type of outcomes study, patients or family or friends may identify the patient in an article, even if minimal patient demographic data are presented, such as gender and age. Beyond these basic points, it is useful for outcomes managers to discuss the nature and extent of an outcomes management program with their IRB to receive additional guidance on when a particular proposal should be sent to the IRB for approval.

Instrumentation Studies

Researchers have developed instruments to measure patient outcomes that can be used in both outcomes research and outcomes management. For example, Chapter 12 describes the use of the Ferrans and Powers Quality of Life Index (Ferrans & Powers, 1992) in patients who have undergone the Whipple procedure for pancreatic disease. This instrument represents years of research to establish its reliability and validity through ongoing use and evaluation in a variety of patient populations.

Researchers are also needed to create reliable risk adjustment instruments. Risk adjustment involves estimating the extent to which a patient is at risk for a negative outcome, such as death or postoperative infection, when comparing outcomes among patients or among health care institutions. Pincus et al. (1996) noted that aside from short-term instruments used in the critical care setting, such as the Acute Physiology and Chronic Health Evaluation II system, there are few reliable risk adjustment instruments. As a proxy for risk adjustment, outcomes managers frequently examine comorbidities. For example, in Chapter 7, while examining the relationship of selected interventions to postoperative wound infection, the authors also examine the influence of comorbid factors, such as obesity and diabetes. Demographic variables, such as age, gender, and race, and physiologic variables such as severity of illness may also help to predict patient risk for negative outcomes. For a complete review and evaluation of various methods of risk adjustment, see Iezzoni (1997).

ETHICAL ISSUES IN THE SELECTION AND USE OF PATIENT OUTCOMES

The selection of patient outcomes to be managed should keep at the fore the sacred trust that patients place in us as health professionals. Pellegrino and Thomasma (1988) call the obligation that health professionals have to act for the good of the patient "beneficence in trust." The use of outcomes data in a way that subverts the beneficence of the health professional toward the patient is a violation of that trust. For example, a Texas managed care organization used the outcome of pharmacy charges in a manner that challenged physicians' ability to act in their patients' best interest (Moran, 1998). It made physicians personally responsible for 30% of pharmacy charges higher than the budgeted amount while allowing them to keep 49% of pharmacy charges lower than the budgeted amount. Doctors who had many healthy patients fared well, but those with very sick patients were significantly penalized. Moran noted that this misuse of patient outcomes data could potentially harm chronically ill patients by making care more difficult to obtain.

Another misuse of patient outcomes is the denial of needed care to groups of patients based on severity of illness or payer status. When Detroit's Henry Ford Health System was losing money on its 40,000 Medicaid patients, some suggested eliminating the Medicaid patients from the system. Others objected, however, noting that abandoning these patients was inconsistent with the mission of the health system. Ultimately, the Medicaid patients remained (Pasternack, 1998).

Part I of this book describes how to begin to measure patient outcomes. Identifying outcomes, selecting instruments to measure outcomes, and the collection, analysis, and presentation of outcomes data are detailed in separate chapters. Part II of the book includes eight clinical chapters that serve as examples of outcomes measurement. Each of the clinical chapters is divided into eight sections that lead the reader through the process of measuring outcomes in a particular group of patients:

- Identifying the patient outcome
- Building the team
- Selecting an instrument
- Measuring the patient outcome
- Analyzing the data
- Summarizing the findings
- Applying the findings to practice
- Planning future patient outcomes projects

The person who possesses patient outcomes data and presents it well can inspire others to participate in its interpretation. The management of patient outcomes data described in this book will assist the reader to promote a multidisciplinary approach that is empowering to all members of the health team. This power, when placed in the service of the patient, can guide the images we create, the outcomes we achieve, and the restoration of patient trust.

REFERENCES

Agency for Health Care Policy and Research. (1998). Available: http://www.ahcpr.gov/data/94drga.htm.

Brooten, D., & Naylor, M. D. (1995). Nurses' effect on changing patient outcomes. *Image—The Journal of Nursing Scholarship, 27*(2), 95-99.

Epstein, R. S., & Sherwood, L. M. (1996). From outcomes research to disease management: A guide for the perplexed. *Annals of Internal Medicine, 124,* 832-837.

Erickson, S. M. (1998). The Vanderbilt model of outcomes management. *Critical Care Nursing Clinics of North America, 10,* 13-20.

Ferrans, C., & Powers, M. (1992). Psychometric assessment of the Quality of Life Index. *Research in Nursing and Health, 15,* 111-119.

Freudenheim, M. (1998, September 29). (Loosely) managed care is in demand. *New York Times,* pp. C1, C3.

Greene, J. (1997). Has managed care lost its soul? *Hospitals & Health Networks, 71,* 36-40.

Harris, M. D. (1991). Clinical and financial outcomes in patient care in a home health care agency. *Journal of Nursing Quality Assurance, 5,* 106.

Hegyvary, S. T. (1991). Issues in outcomes research. *Journal of Nursing Quality Assurance, 5,* 1-6.

Iezzoni, L. I. (1997). The risks of risk adjustment. *Journal of the American Medical Association, 278,* 1600-1607.

Jennings, B. M. (1991). Patient outcomes research: Seizing the opportunity. *Advances in Nursing Science, 14,* 59-72.

Lagoe, R. J., & Aspling, D. L. (1997). Benchmarking and clinical pathway implementation on a multihospital basis. *Nursing Economics, 15*(3), 131-137.

Lasker-Hertz, S., & Houston, S. (1995). Facilitating outcomes research. *Nurse Investigator, 2,* 1-2.

Moran, T. M. (1998). Cow town showdown. *Texas Medicine, 94,* 40-41.

Pasternack, A. (1998). Information underload. *Hospitals & Health Networks, 72,* 28-30.

Pellegrino, E., & Thomasma, D. (1988). *For the patient's good.* New York: Oxford University Press.

Pincus, H. A., Zarin, D. A., & West, J. C. (1996). Peering into the "black box." Measuring the outcomes of managed care. *Archives in General Psychiatry, 53,* 870-877.

Porter, J. E. (1995). The benchmarking effort for networking children's hospitals (BENCHmark). *Journal on Quality Improvement, 21,* 395-406.

CHAPTER 2

Selection of Instruments to Measure Outcomes and Planning for Data Management

Victoria Mock

Marie T. Nolan

Once the outcomes of interest have been identified, the next important step is to select appropriate instruments and to develop a careful plan to manage the outcomes data.

SELECTION OF INSTRUMENTS TO MEASURE OUTCOMES

Selecting an instrument to measure outcomes of interest is an essential and often challenging process. It includes considering the theoretical or conceptual definition of the outcome being measured, identifying appropriate instruments and methods for measuring the outcome, locating and acquiring the instruments and administering and scoring them, and evaluating instrument quality, reliability, and validity (Waltz, Strickland, & Lenz, 1991).

The way in which a specific outcome variable is defined should guide the selection of instruments to measure the outcome. For example, if the conceptual definition of *fatigue* is a "self-perceived state," then it should be measured on a

13

self-report instrument, such as a rating scale or visual analog scale. If *fatigue* is defined as a decreased ability to perform physical work, this outcome should be measured by an appropriate test of physical functioning, such as treadmill performance or the 12-minute walk test. Furthermore, consideration should be given to the purpose for which the researcher will use an instrument compared to the purpose for which the instrument was originally developed. A symptom checklist developed for screening clinical populations may not be suitable for measuring effects of an intervention to decrease specific side effects of treatment when more comprehensive symptom information is desirable.

Case managers, graduate students, and staff members often consult nurse researchers for help in identifying and locating appropriate instruments to measure specific outcomes. One useful and easy method to identify tools for an outcome of interest is to review the literature on the topic being studied and learn how other investigators have measured the outcome. Usually, journal articles include some information about the reliability, validity, and general performance of instruments used in the research being reported. A review of the literature on a specific outcome may also reveal published methodological articles on specific instrument development and testing in the field. In addition, a few books have been devoted to evaluating instruments to measure health care outcomes. A recent, comprehensive volume by Frank-Stromborg and Olsen (1997), *Instruments for Clinical Health-Care Research,* reviews hundreds of instruments that measure specific health-related variables. Another useful reference is *Measuring Health—A Guide to Rating Scales and Questionnaires* by McDowell and Newell (1996). Computerized databases of research instruments are the most recent development in the effort to facilitate identifying and locating appropriate measurement tools.

A variety of instruments and methods of administration are available to measure outcomes of care. Many instruments used to measure outcomes of interest to nursing are self-report questionnaires or scales, such as Likert scales, symptom checklists, visual analog scales, or numeric rating scales (e.g., pain measured on a 0 to 10 scale). Self-report data can also be obtained by structured or unstructured focus groups or interviews that are tape-recorded and transcribed to written format or simply hand-recorded by an interviewer as the subject responds to questions.

Observational methods are also often used in measuring and recording outcomes. Common examples include the functional status of patients, staging of wounds, crying behaviors of toddlers, responsiveness of newborns, and confusion in the elderly. Subject behaviors are rated and categorized or described using a structured procedure and format.

Selection of instruments also involves a careful consideration of their sensitivity, selectivity, appropriateness for the subject population, and feasibility. Sensitivity is the ability of an instrument to reflect small differences or changes in the characteristic being measured. Sensitivity is particularly important when an outcome is being measured repeatedly in the same subjects over time, when experimental and standard conditions are not very different, and when physiologic measurements are used (Stewart & Archbold, 1992, 1993). Selectivity reflects an instrument's ability to correctly identify a variable or outcome being studied and to distinguish it from similar variables—for example, distinguishing "fatigue" from "weakness." Appropriateness refers to factors such as age, reading level, cultural congruence, and illness acuity. Children, the elderly, and very ill patients may have difficulty completing questionnaires. In these situations, interviews or observational measurements may be preferable, or research assistants may be hired and trained to help with questionnaire completion.

The feasibility of an instrument refers to its cost, time and ease of administration and scoring, and its acceptability to patients. The most desirable instruments are brief, easy to understand and administer, inexpensive, and able to be scanned into a computer database (see Chapter 6, this volume).

Nurses new to outcomes management often make the mistake of collecting much more data than are needed, thinking that it may be helpful later or provide additional interesting information. The obvious hazard is a significant burden to patients who participate or to the staff who collect, enter, and analyze the data. This can lead to a higher drop-out rate (especially for the acutely ill) and burnout for staff as well as an accumulation of much data that are never used. Careful planning in the early stage of an outcomes project can limit burden to subjects and facilitate maximum use of resources to complete the project.

Obtaining a copy of the tool and permission to use it are the next steps in the process. Instruments are considered the intellectual property of their authors or creators and are generally copyrighted. If the entire instrument has been published in a noncopyrighted journal or is in the public domain, then it may be used without permission (with a citation of the journal)—unless a footnote indicates the instrument is copyrighted or there is a copyright or trademark symbol (© or ™). If the instrument is copyrighted or not published in its entirety, the author or publisher must be contacted for written permission to use the tool, information on scoring, and to obtain a full copy of the instrument. An instrument may never be altered or adapted without permission. It is useful to identify the tool developer and his or her affiliated institution from a recent publication and write or call as an initial contact. Ask for a forwarding address if the author has left the institution. There is often a charge to use an instrument, and the author may ask you to send the results of your project when it is completed. This can help the developer to improve the tool. Many instruments are commercially available (with an accompanying manual) and may be purchased by qualified researchers (Jacobson, 1997). In this book, several of the clinical chapters include a copy of the instrument(s) used in the particular study described (reprinted with permission).

EVALUATING INSTRUMENT QUALITY

The researcher's ability to accurately answer the research question depends mostly on the quality of instruments and methods used in the project. Instruments can never measure a variable or outcome perfectly (a true score); they include some random and systematic error. Chance variations in subjects (e.g., the presence of pain) or conditions of data collection (e.g., varying settings) result in random error, whereas systematic error results from a consistent factor that affects all measurements made with the instrument (e.g., a scale that weighs 5 pounds more than true weight). The goal of measurement is to maximize accuracy of scores by minimizing measurement error. The fundamental characteristics of quality in an instrument are its reliability and validity.

Reliability

Reliability, the most basic characteristic, involves the consistency or repeatability of measurements with the instrument. A newborn weighed by two nurses (or by one nurse on two consecutive attempts) will weigh the same each time if the scales are reliable. Reliability is generally evaluated in terms of stability, internal consistency, and equivalence. Assessment of stability involves test-retest procedures, administering the same instrument to a sample of subjects on two occasions (typically 2 to 4 weeks apart), and comparing the scores in a correlation procedure. The resulting correlation coefficient may range from −1.00 to 1.00; scores higher than .70 are considered satisfactory. This approach should not be used when the outcome being measured would be expected to change over time (e.g., pain, anxiety, or functional status). Reliability as equivalence involves comparing the observations of two or more observers for interrater reliability. For example, if crying behavior of infants is rated on a scale of 0 to 4 by two different observers working independently, the scores can be correlated to determine interrater reliability. A value of .90 or higher is desirable, and a value lower than .80 should cause concern about reliability (Burns & Grove, 1997).

The most widely used approach to reliability is internal consistency measured by Cronbach's alpha coefficient. An instrument is internally consistent to the degree that its items measure the same construct. For example, a questionnaire on pain will have high internal consistency if all the questions refer to aspects of pain. If several questions on past medical history are included, these could not be assumed to correlate with pain and probably would lower the Cronbach's alpha. A coefficient of .80 or higher is expected for an established instrument, although .70 is acceptable for an instrument under development. Whether one uses a standard instrument or develops a new one, reliability should be determined for each administration of an instrument to a group of subjects because reliability changes with each administration (Polit & Hungler, 1999).

Validity

Validity reflects the degree to which an instrument measures what it is supposed to measure. A clinician measuring depression needs to use an instrument that clearly differentiates depression from fatigue or unmanaged pain. Assessment of instrument validity encompasses content validity, criterion-related validity, and construct validity. Content validity is based on the judgments of experts in the subject matter and is concerned with whether the test items accurately and comprehensively measure the content area.

Criterion-related validity refers to the correlation between a measure and some outside indicator of the attribute being measured—for example, the correlation between self-reported pain and requests for pain medication. There are two types of criterion-related validity—concurrent validity and predictive validity. Concurrent validity refers to the current condition in relation to an identified criterion, whereas predictive validity refers to predicting performance on some future criterion such as the probability of falls predicted from mental status scores.

Construct validity focuses on the attribute or concept being measured and its theoretical meaning. One approach to construct validity is the known-groups technique. In this procedure, the instrument is administered to two groups known to be high and low on the attribute measured. For example, a new instrument to measure pain might be used when patients request analgesia and 1 hour after their pain medication is received. Other ways to determine construct validity are factor analysis and multitrait-multimethod procedures. These more complex procedures may require help from a nurse researcher or a statistician.

High reliability and validity are essential characteristics of instruments used to measure patient outcomes. Only when these are ensured can the project team have confidence that the data collected accurately reflect the patient experience. High reliability and validity are more likely when the team uses standardized instruments that have been used widely in the selected patient population. Standardized instruments have the additional advantage of availability of normative data with which to compare the study sample data.

Reliability and Validity in Biophysiologic Measures

Physiologic variables, such as blood pressure, vital capacity, or weight, are often selected as significant outcomes of care. Physiologic measures may include laboratory biochemical measurements (arterial blood gases and serum potassium), physical measurements (body weight and urinary output), and microbiologic measurements (colonies of bacteria). Threats to the reliability and validity (referred to as precision and accuracy) of biophysiologic measurements include problems with the instrument or equipment and human error in the measurement process. Precision can be increased by taking repeated measures (e.g., three blood pressure readings) and averaging the values.

Calibration procedures on instruments are used to improve accuracy of measurements (DeKeyser & Pugh, 1997). Laboratory procedures can also be evaluated for their accuracy and precision. The quality of all data, biophysiologic and psychosocial, is only as good as the instruments and procedures that are used to obtain the data.

DEVELOPING INSTRUMENTS

Sometimes well-tested instruments are not available to measure an outcome of interest and developing an instrument is the best alternative. Chapter 9 reports a study of postprostatectomy incontinence with an instrument developed for the project because no appropriate tool was available. Such a step should be undertaken only after an extensive search of the literature has been performed and advice from researchers knowledgeable in the area has been obtained. Although instrument creation can be a time-consuming and complex effort, simple instruments modeled after standardized tools can be developed by case managers using basic principles with the consultation of someone experienced in the process. The plan of the outcomes project should include realistic additional time if an instrument for the study is to be developed and tested.

If demographic or health outcome instruments need to be developed for the project, a review of similar forms from other projects can save much time and energy. Visual analog scales and numeric rating scales often can be adapted; for example, the standard 0 to 10 scale used to measure pain level has also been used to report fatigue, nausea, and other symptoms. Developing an entire questionnaire (e.g., to measure incontinence) is more challenging, and an expert in instrument development can be a helpful consultant. Reliability, validity, and other evaluation is required for newly developed instruments.

Even if standardized instruments are selected for an outcomes project, pretesting the tools with a few volunteers from the patient population can be very helpful in evaluating the tool's feasibility and appropriateness. It is also helpful to determine how long it takes subjects to complete the instruments. Although pretesting requires additional time before the study begins, it can save time and contribute to more accurate measurement of outcomes in the end. For example, during pretesting of a visual analog scale to measure body image in women treated for breast cancer, some subjects interpreted satisfaction with body to refer to one's "nude" body, and others understood it to mean one's "clothed" body. The instrument was modified before use in the final study.

Conducting a pilot of the entire research procedure with 10 or more subjects from the patient population can be an extremely useful component of an outcomes project. Experienced outcomes managers would never consider launching a study without piloting the instruments and procedures. The reward is well worth the time and resources spent in facilitating the smooth and successful conduct of any outcomes project.

PLANNING FOR DATA MANAGEMENT

Once instruments to measure the outcomes of interest have been selected, the next task is to plan for the management of the outcomes data. Sources of existing data need to be examined to avoid duplication of effort in the data collection process. The format of the data and where the data will reside and what other personnel will be involved in the management of the data are important issues to address at the outset.

Data Sources

The first step in planning for patient outcomes data management is to explore all existing sources of data. Pasternack (1998) described a hospital that assigned two groups the task of improving the care of patients with asthma. Both groups decided to start by determining the age range and distribution of the asthma patients treated at the hospital. One group reviewed 3 months of patient records to accomplish this task. The other group simply asked the hospital's information systems department to pull the data from a year's worth of computerized patient records. Using existing data sets can increase the ease and efficiency of measuring patient outcomes. It is also important to consider the accuracy and reliability of each database used.

An organization may have many types of patient data drawn from flowcharts, medical records, critical pathways, and financial reports (Jones, 1993). In the best possible situation, these data reside in a single data warehouse and are easily accessible to data users. In the worst situation, data are scattered among multiple networks and personal computers (PCs) requiring users to search, collect, and piece together a usable database. Whatever the state of the organization's information system, it is worthwhile to explore all existing data sources to avoid unnecessary data collection and entry.

One source of patient outcomes data in the acute care setting is the hospital discharge database. This type of database has been criticized, however, for its high degree of inaccuracy. One source of the inaccuracy is related to the omission of information from the medical records that serve as the source for the coding of diagnoses and procedures. Another source of error occurs when data in the records are misinterpreted by coders (Wray et al., 1995). When used in combination with other institutional data sources, however, errors in documentation and coding can be identified and minimized. Wray et al. suggested viewing the discharge database as an "imperfect compass" that can be used to direct us toward possible opportunities for improvement in the quality of care.

Data Formats

When planning to measure patient outcomes within a specialty area, it may be necessary to create new data sets to explore specialty-specific outcomes. Most of the case study chapters in this book describe outcomes projects that required the creation of new databases. Before an individual outcomes manager creates a new database, it is useful to plan with the organization's information systems department how the new database can be integrated into existing databases. Another important consideration is the ease with which the data can be imported into the statistical analysis program the outcomes manager will use to analyze the patient outcomes data.

Database Management and Personnel

A very important part of planning outcomes management includes identifying where the database for a particular patient outcomes project will reside. The data may have been pulled from a variety of sources, with perhaps the addition of new data collected specifically for the outcomes project. Placing the data on a server would allow multiple members of the multidisciplinary team to access the data but would require careful planning with regard to who could or could not enter, edit, or delete data to protect the integrity of the data. In contrast, placing the data on the PC of one of the team members could offer greater protection from corruption of the data file but would not provide members with the same degree of accessibility. Regardless of where the data reside, issues of security should be discussed at the outset to safeguard both the confidentiality of the patient information and the integrity of the data. There are multiple strategies to secure confidential patient data that can be discussed with information service experts within the organization (Lawrence, 1994). Efforts to preserve the integrity of the data should include a schedule for backing up data should there be a system failure that corrupts or deletes the data.

A critical component of measuring patient outcomes is planning for the personnel who will be responsible for each phase of the data management process. The major steps involved in the management of patient outcomes data include

- Deciding on valid, reliable instruments for measuring specific outcomes

- Obtaining data from existing sources

- Collecting additional data

- Entering data

- Merging data from various sources with the new data

- Maintaining the data

- Analyzing the data, creating graphics, and presenting the results

The level of support provided for each step of the management of the patient outcomes data will depend on an organization's resources. The final step involving the analysis and presentation of data, however, involves skills that are fast becoming entry-level skills for those who manage patient outcomes. One reason for this is that data analysis is often a process and not an event in outcomes management. When the multidisciplinary team examines the first round of data analysis, new questions may be generated that require additional analysis. Having to wait for data to be analyzed centrally by nonclinicians can be a source of delay that causes the team to lose momentum. Moreover, the success of the outcomes manager is often related to his or her ability to serve as leader in the multidisciplinary group. Having the results of the data analysis in advance of the rest of the group allows the outcomes manager time to examine the information, anticipate concerns, and develop possible courses of action for the group to consider.

Erickson (1998) described the evolution of the case management program at Vanderbilt University Medical Center. One of the important components of the Vanderbilt program was the training of case managers in the management and analysis of data. Other case management programs throughout the country are reaching similar conclusions. Data management and analysis skills are essential for those who are responsible for managing patient outcomes.

These are exciting times for those managing patient outcomes. Information technology has never been more advanced, the cooperation among health professionals has never been better, and the chance to make significant improvements in the care processes has never been greater. Our success in achieving the best possible outcomes may rest with the leaders who have the skill to bring all the previously discussed factors together in a unified vision for patient care.

REFERENCES

Burns, N., & Grove, S. K. (1997). *The practice of nursing research: Conduct, critique, & utilization* (3rd ed.). Philadelphia: Saunders.

DeKeyser, F. G., & Pugh, L. C. (1997). Physiologic measurements. In M. Frank-Stromborg & S. Olsen (Eds.), *Instruments for clinical health-care research* (2nd ed., pp. 3-19). Sudbury, MA: Jones & Bartlett.

Erickson, S. M. (1998). The Vanderbilt model of outcomes management. *Critical Care Nursing Clinics of North America, 10,* 13-20.

Frank-Stromborg, M., & Olsen, S. (1997). *Instruments for clinical health-care research* (2nd ed.). Sudbury, MA: Jones & Bartlett.

Jacobson, S. F. (1997). Evaluating instruments for use in clinical nursing research. In M. Frank-Stromborg & S. Olsen (Eds.), *Instruments for clinical health-care research* (2nd ed., pp. 3-19). Sudbury, MA: Jones & Bartlett.

Jones, K. R. (1993). Outcomes analysis: Methods and issues. *Nursing Economics, 11,* 145-152.

Lawrence, L. M. (1994). Safeguarding the confidentiality of automated medical information. *Journal of Quality Improvement, 20,* 639-646.

McDowell, I., & Newell, C. (1996). *Measuring health—A guide to rating scales and questionnaires* (2nd ed.). New York: Oxford University Press.

Pasternack, A. (1998). Information underload. *Hospitals & Health Networks, 72,* 28-30.

Polit, D. F., & Hungler, B. P. (1999). *Nursing research: Principles and methods* (6th ed.). Philadelphia: J. B. Lippincott.

Stewart, B. J., & Archbold, P. G. (1992). Focus on psychometrics—Nursing intervention studies require outcome measures that are sensitive to change: Part 1. *Research in Nursing & Health, 15,* 477-481.

Stewart, B. J., & Archbold, P. G. (1993). Focus on psychometrics—Nursing intervention studies require outcome measures that are sensitive to change: Part 2. *Research in Nursing & Health, 16,* 77-81.

Waltz, C. F., Strickland, O. L., & Lenz, E. R. (1991). *Measurement in nursing research* (2nd ed.). Philadelphia: F. A. Davis.

Wray, N. P., Ashton, C. M., Kuykendall, D. H., Petersen, N. J., Souchek, J., & Hollingsworth, J. C. (1995). Selecting disease-outcome pairs for monitoring the quality of hospital care. *Medical Care, 33,* 75-89.

CHAPTER 3

Creation and Manipulation of SPSS Data Files

Marie T. Nolan

The ability to create data files that can then be used to measure patient outcomes is a tremendously powerful skill. The goal of this chapter is to enable the reader who has little or no data management experience to create patient data files and manipulate the data in these files using SPSS Version 9.0 (1999). By following the instructions in this chapter, the reader will first create a data file named *cvpts.sav* that contains data on cardiovascular patients. The reader will save this file and create a new file named *ptsat.sav* that contains data on patient satisfaction. Finally, the reader will learn how to import data from spreadsheets such as Microsoft Excel (1997) or from relational databases such as Microsoft Access (1997).

Data files can be created from the beginning or imported from a variety of other programs. In addition, there are many interesting ways to manipulate SPSS data files when examining patient outcomes. For example, imagine that your institution is considering developing a cardiovascular health program for women. If you have a file with data from all cardiovascular patients in your institution, you can select out the data on women to analyze. It will then take only a moment to determine the high-frequency causes for admission, procedures during hospitalization, and the mean age and length of stay for the women in this data file. Manipulating data can also mean using the data to perform calculations. For example, if you have a data file with patient admission and discharge dates, SPSS will allow you to subtract the admission date from the

23

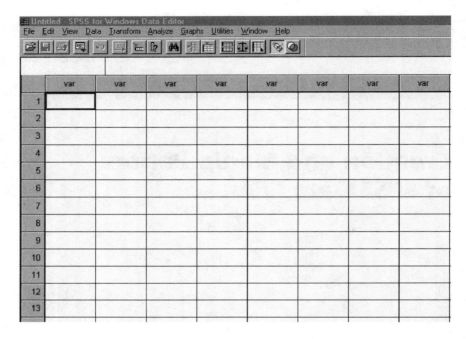

Figure 3.1. *Data Editor* (Reproduced With Permission of SPSS, Inc.)

discharge date to create a new variable that you could label "los" for length of stay. After mastering the essential SPSS skills in data management presented here, it is recommended that the reader consult the more advanced literature on using SPSS listed under Further Reading.

CREATING AN SPSS DATA FILE

When working in SPSS, you will primarily be working in the *Data Editor* or the *Viewer*. The *Data Editor* displays the data with which you are working, and the *Viewer* displays the results of data analysis or graphics created to summarize the data. Most of this chapter will involve working in the *Data Editor*. To begin, after clicking on the SPSS icon to open the SPSS program, the first screen to appear is the *Data Editor*. This looks like an empty grid or spreadsheet (Figure 3.1).

Creating a Numeric Variable

Generally, when using SPSS to manage patient information, rows will represent patients and columns will represent variables such as age, gender, cost, and

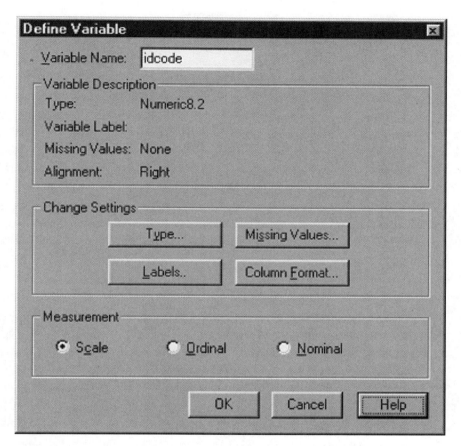

Figure 3.2. *Define Variable* Dialog Box (Reproduced With Permission of SPSS, Inc.)

length of stay. To create the first variable, double click on the first gray box labeled *var.* This will bring up the *Define Variable* dialog box (Figure 3.2).

Notice that the variable name is *VAR00001.* SPSS automatically assigns a number to each variable. You can change this to a variable name of your choice, but the name must begin with a letter, be less than eight characters, and contain no blank spaces. Consider this a short name or "nickname" for the variable. To change *VAR00001* to a variable name of your choice, type the variable name *idcode,* for example, in the white box next to the words *Variable Name.* When dealing with patient data, it is useful to assign patients an identification code, such as a medical record number, that will allow for tracking the data back to its original source. The *Define Variable* dialog box also gives a brief description of the variable. SPSS assumes that the variable is a numeric variable unless you

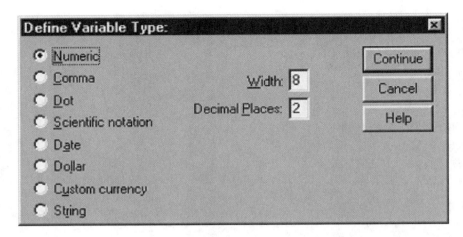

Figure 3.3. *Define Variable Type* Dialog Box (Reproduced With Permission of SPSS, Inc.)

indicate otherwise. For example, in the *Define Variable* dialog box that you are currently in, click on the small gray box labeled *Type* . . . This will bring up the dialog box, *Define Variable Type* (Figure 3.3).

The darkened circle next to the word *Numeric* indicates that this variable is a number. Other commonly used variable types are *Date, Dollar,* and *String. String* means that the variable uses letters rather than numbers. A patient's name is an example of a *String* variable. Also in the *Define Variable Type* dialog box is the width of the variable and the decimal places allowed in this variable. SPSS automatically assigns a width of 8 characters and two decimal places. You can change these numbers. For example, to change the width of the variable to 25 characters to allow for larger numbers (or longer names when entering string variables), just click on the white box next to the word *Width* and enter the number 25. This will replace the number 8 in the *Width* box. Select the gray button *Continue* to return to the *Define Variable* dialog box. In the *Define Variable* dialog box, notice that in the *Variable Description* box, you can see that the space next to the words *Variable Label* is blank. The *Variable Label* is the full name for your variable that will appear next to the variable on your data printouts when you analyze data and on your graphics if you use this variable to create a graphic such as a pie chart or bar chart. To create a variable label, click on the gray box with the word *Labels.* In the white box next to the words *Variable Label,* enter a label such as *ID Code.* Then click on the box *Continue* and then click on the box *OK* to return to the *Data Editor.* You should now see the label *idcode* inside the gray box at the top of column 1 in the *Data Editor.* Congratulations. You have created your first variable in the data file.

Creating a String Variable

Creating a string variable is similar to creating a numeric variable except that because SPSS begins by assuming that all variables are numeric, you will have to indicate when you are dealing with letters or words instead of numbers. Begin in the *Data Editor* by double clicking on the next gray box with the label *var.* This will bring up the *Define Variable* dialog box. Begin by typing *lastname* in the white box next to the words *Variable Name.* (Hint: Did you remember that there are no spaces in variable names?) Next, click on the gray box labeled *Type.* This brings up the *Define Variable Type* dialog box. Next, click on the word *String* to select this as the variable type. Then, in the white box next to the word *Characters,* delete the 8 and replace it with 25. This will allow you the extra width that you will need when entering names. Next, click *Continue* to get back to the *Define Variable* dialog box. Click on the gray box named *Labels* to bring up the *Define Labels* dialog box. Enter the words *Last Name* in the white box next to the words *Variable Label.* Because this is the variable label and not the variable name, you can insert spaces between words. Next, click on the gray box labeled *Continue,* and then click on the gray box labeled *OK.* This returns you to the *Data Editor,* in which you can see your new string variable, *lastname.*

Creating Value Labels

Assigning numeric values to some categorical variables can make data entry more efficient because one need only enter a single number rather than an entire word. For example, with the variable gender, the number 1 can be used to indicate male, and the number 2 can be used to indicate female. For a variable representing satisfaction with postoperative pain management, 1 can mean very dissatisfied, 2 can mean dissatisfied, 3 can mean satisfied, and 4 can mean very satisfied.

Beginning again from the *Data Editor,* double click on a gray box containing the letters *var.* This brings up the *Define Variable* dialog box. In the white box labeled *Variable Name,* enter the word *gender.* Next, click on the gray box with the word *Labels* inside it. This will bring up the *Define Labels* dialog box (Figure 3.4).

Enter the word *Gender* in the white box next to the words *Variable Label.* Next, enter the number 1 in the white box next to the word *Value.* Then enter the word *male* in the white box next to the words *Value Label.* Then click on the gray box with the word *Add* inside it. Now you should see *1 = "male"* inside the white box at the bottom of the *Define Labels* dialog box. Next, enter the number 2 in the white box next to the word *Value.* Then enter the word *female* in the white box next to the words *Value Label.* Then click on the gray box with

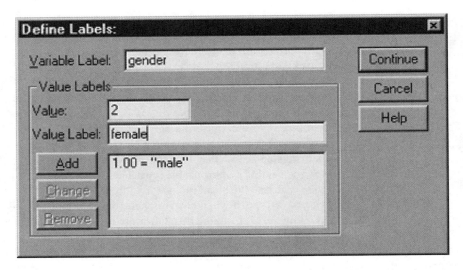

Figure 3.4. *Define Labels* Dialog Box (Reproduced With Permission of SPSS, Inc.)

the word *Add* inside it. Now you should see *2 = "female"* inside the white box at the bottom of the *Define Labels* dialog box. Then click on *Continue,* and then click on *OK.* This will bring you back to the *Data Editor,* in which you should see the word gender at the top of one of the variable columns.

Creating Date Variables

SPSS has several options for defining date as a variable. From the *Data Editor,* double click on a gray box with *var* inside. Type the word *admitdat* in the white box next to the words *Variable Name.* Next, click on the gray box with the word *Labels* on it. This brings up the *Define Labels* dialog box. Enter the words *Admit Date* in the white box next to the words *Variable Label.* Then click on *Continue.* Now, click on the gray box with the word *Type* on it. This will bring up the *Define Variable Type* dialog box. Click on the word *Date* and notice that this opens a white box to the right with several date format options from which to choose. For example, if you prefer to state a date as 10/11/99, you would select the date option *mmddyy.* (This allows you two numbers for the month followed by two numbers for the day and two numbers for the year.) Next, click *Continue* and then *OK.* You should see the word *admitdat* at the top of one of the variable columns. You have successfully defined your admission date variable. Repeat this process to define a discharge date called *dcdat.*

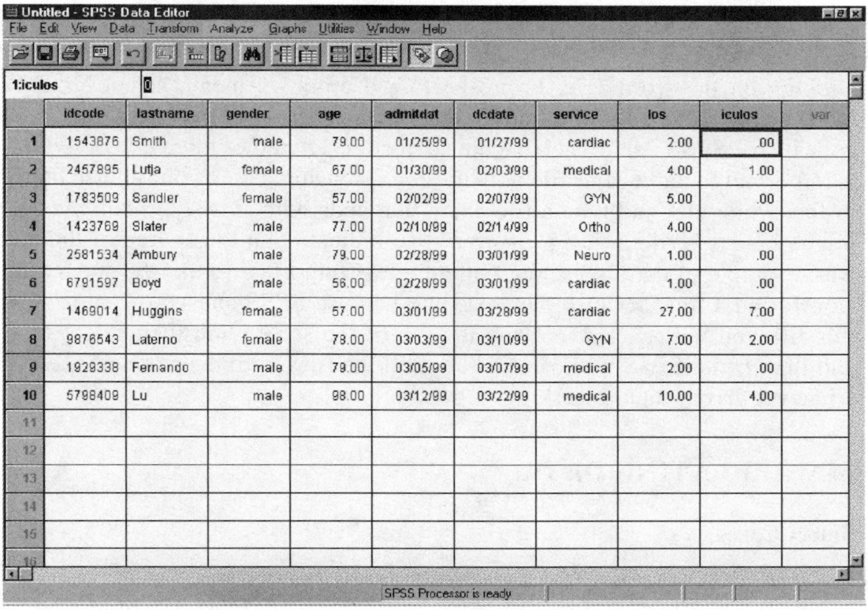

	idcode	lastname	gender	age	admitdat	dcdate	service	los	iculos	var
1	1543876	Smith	male	79.00	01/25/99	01/27/99	cardiac	2.00	.00	
2	2457895	Lutja	female	67.00	01/30/99	02/03/99	medical	4.00	1.00	
3	1783509	Sandler	female	57.00	02/02/99	02/07/99	GYN	5.00	.00	
4	1423769	Slater	male	77.00	02/10/99	02/14/99	Ortho	4.00	.00	
5	2581534	Ambury	male	79.00	02/28/99	03/01/99	Neuro	1.00	.00	
6	6791597	Boyd	male	56.00	02/28/99	03/01/99	cardiac	1.00	.00	
7	1469014	Huggins	female	57.00	03/01/99	03/28/99	cardiac	27.00	7.00	
8	9876543	Laterno	female	78.00	03/03/99	03/10/99	GYN	7.00	2.00	
9	1929338	Fernando	male	79.00	03/05/99	03/07/99	medical	2.00	.00	
10	5798409	Lu	male	98.00	03/12/99	03/22/99	medical	10.00	4.00	
11										
12										
13										
14										
15										
16										

Figure 3.5. Data Editor With Data for 10 Hypothetical Patients (Reproduced With Permission of SPSS, Inc.)

ENTERING DATA

Now that you have defined several variables, you are ready to enter data. When entering patient data, it is often most convenient to enter data by row rather than by column. This means that you would enter all the data on one patient before entering data on the next patient. To practice this, begin with the *Data Editor* that includes the variables you have created: *idcode, lastname, gender, admitdat,* and *dcdat.* Click your left mouse button on the first white box in row 1, column 1. Enter the number 1. Now, use the right arrow key on your keyboard to arrow one space to the right and enter a last name (remember that you defined this as 25 characters, so if you enter a name with more than 25 letters you will have to redefine the variable width). Arrow over one space to the right, and enter a 1 or 2 for gender. Next, arrow one space to the right, and enter a date using the format mmddyy. To return to the next row, you can either arrow back to the left one space at a time or just click on the gray box at the beginning of row 2. This will automatically bring you to the beginning of row 2 and will highlight the entire row. To begin entering data for row 2, just click on the first white box in row 2, column 1. Enter data for all the variables for 10 rows (Figure 3.5).

Important: Remember to save the file after entering data for every few patients. You can do this by going to the menu at the top of your screen and clicking on the word *File*. From the *File* drop-down menu, select *Save As*. Notice that in the white box under the words *File Name* the characters *.sav* appear. All SPSS data files have the extension .sav rather than .doc or .wpd. It is important to name your file with the *sav* extension. Click your mouse button in this white box and type a file name that ends with .sav. For example, you might save this file as *CV Patients.sav* to indicate that the source of the data was a sample of cardiovascular patients. It is important to use the .sav extension for data files because the next time you use SPSS and you want to open this file you will click *File* from the top of the screen and then select *Open* and then *Data*. SPSS will offer a list of all the files with the extension .sav in whatever drive you are working.

MANIPULATING DATA

Select Cases

The SPSS allows you to separate your data in many ways. Perhaps you have a patient data file with men and women and you would just like to look at the outcomes for women. Also, there may be a data set that includes both children and adults and you would like to just examine the data for the children. You can do this by using the *Select Cases* option in SPSS. For example, you can select out the women in the file *cvpts.sav* that you have just created. Beginning at the *Data Editor* of this file, click on the word *Data* at the top of your screen. This will drop down the *Data* menu. From this menu, click on the words *Select Cases*. In the *Select Cases* dialog box that appears, click on the white circle next to the words *If condition is satisfied*. Next, click on the gray box with the word *If* on it. This will bring up the *Select Cases If* dialog box (Figure 3.6).

In the box at the left that contains the names of the variables in your file, double click on the variable *gender*. This will move the word gender into the empty box at the right. Next, click on the equals (=) sign on the keypad. This will bring the = sign into the box to the right of gender. Next, click on the number 2 from the keypad. This will bring the number 2 into the box above the keypad so that inside the box you will see *gender = 2*. Next, click *Continue* in the gray box below the keypad, and then click *OK*. This will bring you back to the *Data Editor,* in which you will notice that the row number in the gray box at the beginning of each row is still visible for all rows but has been crossed out for the rows with male patients. Any analysis you do at this point will be done only on women patients.

Important: When you are finished analyzing the data on women and wish to return to the entire data base including men, click on the word *Data* at the

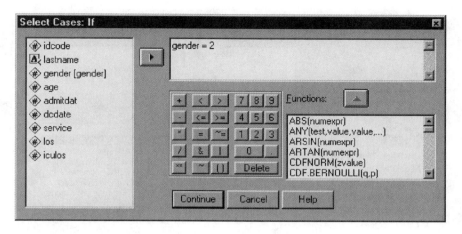

Figure 3.6. *Select Cases If* Dialog Box (Reproduced With Permission of SPSS, Inc.)

top of the screen and then click on *Select Cases* in the *Data* menu. This will bring up the *Select Cases* dialog box. Click on the white circle next to the words *All Cases,* and then click on *OK.* The cross-hatching at the beginning of the rows should be gone. Now, all patients in the file are available for analysis.

Perform Calculations

Length of Stay

Length of stay is a common patient outcome of concern. In addition, there may be a variety of other time periods of interest, such as days from surgery to discharge or days from admission to the provision of a particular intervention such as discharge planning or physical therapy. If dates have been formatted according to the procedures outlined in Creating Date Variables, the dates can be used to calculate the time periods of interest. For example, beginning at the *Data Editor* with the file *cvpts.sav* that you just created, click on the word *Transform* at the top of the screen; in the menu box that drops down, click on *Compute.* This brings up the *Compute Variable* dialog box (Figure 3.7)

In the empty white box, under the words *Target Variable,* give the variable a name such as *los* (for length of stay). Next, click on the gray box with the words *Type & Label* on it. This brings up the *Compute Variable: Type and Label* dialog box. In the white box next to the word *Label,* type in a variable label such as *Length of Stay.* Then click *Continue.* In the *Compute Variable* dialog box, go to the white box with several abbreviations under the word *Functions.* The

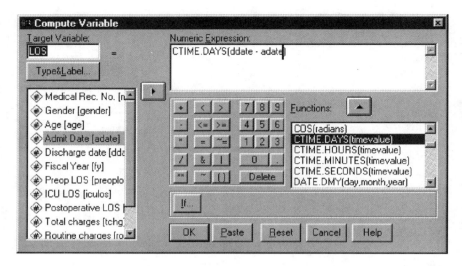

Figure 3.7. *Compute Variable* Dialog Box (Reproduced With Permission of SPSS, Inc.)

abbreviations in this box are listed alphabetically. Using the gray arrow at the right border of the box, scroll down until you reach the abbreviation *CTIME.DAYS(timevalue)*. Double click on this abbreviation to move it up into the empty white box above. You will notice that now the abbreviation reads *CTIME.DAYS(?)*. From the variable list at the left, double click on the variable *ddate*. This will move the variable *ddate* inside the brackets. Next, click on the minus symbol on the keypad below. This will move the minus symbol into the box after the variable *ddate*. Next, return to the variable list and double click on *adate*. This should move *adate* to the box, so that the equation now reads *CTIME.DAYS(ddate-adate)*. Now click *OK*. Your new variable, *los,* will be the last column in your data file.

Scale and Subscale Sums

Patient satisfaction, quality of life, and functional health status are examples of patient outcomes that can be measured using a survey in which the sum of all the survey questions represents the level of the outcome being measured. To demonstrate this, create a new data file by clicking *File,* then *New,* and then *Data.* If SPSS asks if you would like to save changes to your data file *cvpts.sav,* click *Yes* and then continue on to create a new file. Imagine that you have a 10-question patient satisfaction survey with responses that range from 0 ("very dissatisfied") to 4 ("very satisfied"). Create a variable for each question in the survey, and name them sat1 to sat10. Once all 10 variables have been created, enter sample responses for five of the patients.

SPSS will now allow you to calculate the sum of all 10 questions and place this sum in a new variable. To do so, begin from the *Data Editor*. Click on the word *Transform* at the top of the screen, and in the menu box that drops down, click on the word *Compute*. This brings up the *Compute Variable* dialog box. In the empty white box, under the words *Target Variable,* give the variable a name such as *totalsat* (for total satisfaction score). Next, click on the gray box with the words *Type & Label* on it. This brings up the *Compute Variable: Type and Label* dialog box. In the white box next to the word *Label,* type in a variable label such as *Total Satisfaction.* Then click *Continue.* In the *Compute Variable* dialog box, go to the white box with several abbreviations under the word *Functions.* The abbreviations in this box are listed alphabetically. Using the gray arrow at the right border of the box, scroll down until you reach the abbreviation *SUM(numexpr, numexpr...).* Double click on this abbreviation to move it into the empty white box above. Notice how the abbreviation now reads *SUM(?,?).* Next, select the first satisfaction variable, *sat1,* from the variable box at the left, and double click on it. This will move it inside the parentheses of the equation at the right. Place a comma after the first variable, and then double click on the second variable, *sat2,* in the variable box at the right. Place a comma after the second variable. Continue doing this until all the questions in the survey have been moved inside the parentheses. Make sure that you place a comma after every variable except the last variable. Delete any remaining question marks inside the parentheses (Figure 3.8).

Next, click on the gray *OK* button. The new variable, *Totalsat,* will appear at the end of the data file. This same procedure can be used to calculate subscale scores.

Recoding Variables

Sometimes, you may wish to recode variables. This can mean recoding a numeric variable into another numeric variable or recoding a string variable into a numeric variable.

Numeric Variable to Numeric Variable

A commonly recoded numeric patient variable is age. Imagine that you are studying the safety of conscious sedation, and that you have a database of several hundred cases. Using this database, you would like to examine length of time in recovery following sedation by age group. Because older patients may not metabolize the agents given during conscious sedation as readily as

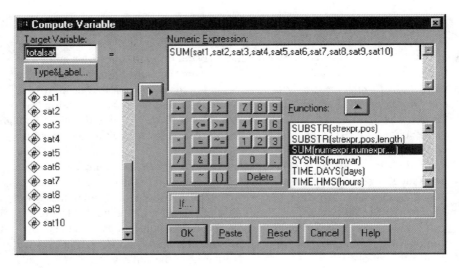

Figure 3.8. *Compute Variable* Dialog Box with Equation for Total Satisfaction Score (Reproduced With Permission of SPSS, Inc.)

younger patients, you may wish to break down the continuous variable of age into the age categories of 18 to 65, 66 to 79, and 80 and older. To do this, go into the *Data Editor* and click on the word *Transform* at the top of the screen. In the menu box that drops down, click on the word *Recode,* and in the menu box that pops up at the right click on the words *Into Different Variables.* In the *Recode Into Different Variables* dialog box that pops up, double click on the variable *age* in the variable box at the left. This will move it to the box on the right. Next, type a variable name and a label in the output variable box at the right. For example, *agecat* could be the variable name and *Age Categories* the variable label. Then click on the gray box labeled *Change.* Next, click on the gray box labeled *Old and New Values.* This brings up the *Recode Into Different Variables: Old and New Values* dialog box. At the left, click on the white circle next to the word *Range.* In the white boxes under the word *Range,* enter the number 18 in the first box and 65 in the second box. On the right side of the dialog box, under the words *New Value,* enter the number 1. Then click on the gray box labeled *Add.* This places the statement *18 thru 65* → *1* in the empty white box. Next, go back to the left of the dialog box, and under the word *Range* enter 66 in the first white box and 79 in the next white box. On the right side of the dialog box, under the words *New Value,* enter the number 2. Then click the gray box labeled *Add.* This places the statement *66 thru 79* → *2 in the white box below. Following the same procedure, make 80 thru 100* → *3* the third statement in the same white box (Figure 3.9).

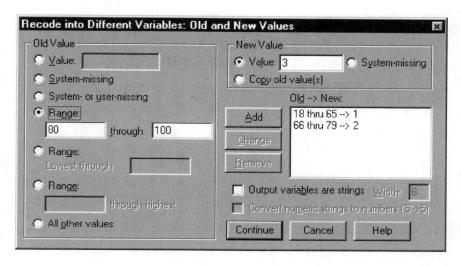

Figure 3.9. *Recode Into Different Variables: Old and New Values* Dialog Box (Reproduced With Permission of SPSS, Inc.)

When this is done, click *Continue* and then click *OK.* At the end of your data file, you will now find a new variable, *agecat,* with the patients' ages recoded into the age categories you just defined. You can use the variable *agecat* as the factor or independent variable in an analysis of variance (ANOVA) procedure comparing the mean time to recovery among the three age categories.

String Variable to Numeric Variable

There are times when you may wish to convert a string variable into a numeric variable. For example, imagine that someone has given you a conscious sedation database to analyze. In this database, the variable indicating the drug administered is a string variable. You decide to compare the time to recovery following the conscious sedation procedure among patients according to the drug they have received. This would require an ANOVA procedure in which the drug would be the factor or independent variable. *Drug* would need to be a numeric variable to carry out this analysis. To convert the string variable *Drug* to a numeric variable, begin in the *Data Editor.* Click on the word *Transform* at the top of the screen. In the menu that drops down, click on *Automatic Recode.* In the *Automatic Recode* dialog box, double click on the variable *drug.* This will move it into the empty box at the right. Next, in the empty white box next to the gray box labeled *New Name,* enter a name such as *drug2* for the new numeric variable to be produced from this string variable. Click on the *New Name* box.

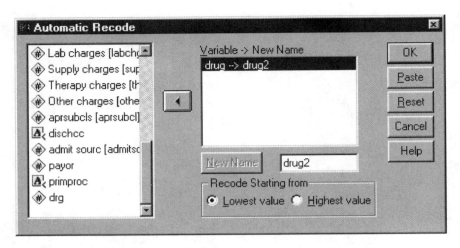

Figure 3.10. *Automatic Recode* Dialog Box (Reproduced With Permission of SPSS, Inc.)

This will move *drug2* into the white box above, which should now contain the phrase *drug* → *drug2* (Figure 3.10).

Then click *OK*. SPSS will assign a number to each drug or drug combination and to any missing data. In this case, 1 = missing data, 2 = Ativan, 3 = Fentanyl, and 4 = Midazolam.

Importing Data Files From Other Programs

When tracking patient outcomes, it may be necessary to import data files that were created in software programs such as Lotus 123 (1997) or Microsoft Excel (1997). To open a file from another program, from the *Data Editor* click *File* and then click *Open.* In the *Open File* dialog box, click on the arrow next to the box labeled *Files of Type.* This will reveal several types of files. Select the file type you are interested in opening (e.g., *Excel*). Then, click on the arrow next to the white box labeled *Look In.* This will reveal available directories for you to select to identify the source of the Excel file. When you have highlighted the directory and name of the file that you would like to open, click the gray box labeled *Open.* This will open the *Opening File Options* dialog box. Click on the white box labeled *Read Variable Names* (Figure 3.11).

It is important to remember to select *Read Variable Names* because it lets SPSS know that the first row in the Excel spreadsheet includes variable names. When importing data from another program, SPSS automatically assigns variable type according to the data in the first row. If you do not select *Read Variable*

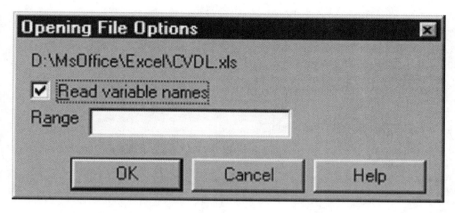

Figure 3.11. *Opening File Options* Dialog Box (Reproduced With Permission of SPSS, Inc.)

Names, SPSS will read the first spreadsheet row as alpha data and will define each variable as a string variable. Once *Read Variable Names* has been selected, click *OK.* This will bring up the file in SPSS. Remember that SPSS accepts variable names that are eight characters or less. If you are importing from a file with variable names that are longer than eight characters, SPSS will automatically truncate the names and bring you to the *Viewer,* in which it will list the truncated variable names. To return to the *Data Editor,* simply click on the grid icon at the top of the screen or click on the word *Windows* at the top of the screen and then click on the name of your data file that will appear in the drop-down menu.

It is important to remember that you must save the file in an SPSS format if you wish it to be in SPSS and not Excel the next time you want to open it. SPSS can also import data from relational databases such as Microsoft Access (1996). To do this, from the *Data Editor* click on *File* and then click on *Database Capture.* Next, click on *New Query* and then highlight the type of file from which you are importing data. Then click on *Next.* From here, follow the instructions on the screen or consult the SPSS manual for more detailed information.

SUMMARY

Measuring patient outcomes requires some basic data management skills. SPSS can be used to create and manipulate data files. This program can accommodate both alpha and numeric variables and can divide data in many ways for analysis. Being able to select out patients of a certain age group or patients who are undergoing a certain treatment is helpful when analyzing the outcomes of selected patient groups.

REFERENCES

Access Version 97 [Computer software]. (1996). Redmond, WA: Microsoft.
Excel Version 97 [Computer software]. (1997). Redmond, WA: Microsoft.
Lotus 123 5.0 [Computer software]. (1997). Cambridge, MA: Lotus Development.
SPSS Version 9.0 [Computer software]. (1999). Chicago: SPSS.

FURTHER READING

Einspruch, E. L. (1998). *An introductory guide to SPSS for Windows*. Thousand Oaks, CA: Sage.
SPSS. (1999). *SPSS Base 9.0*. Chicago: Author.

CHAPTER 4

Overview of Statistical Methods for Measuring Patient Outcomes

Victoria Mock

In the early phases of MEASURING patient outcomes, the analysis of data focuses on the clinical significance of findings with less emphasis on statistical significance. Thus, methods of data analysis—in addition to traditional methods—may involve analyzing change scores, comparing sample data to a standard or benchmark, or using descriptive analyses to identify outliers or variances among patients placed on a critical path. This chapter includes a brief summary of basic measurement concepts and an overview of common statistical methods for measuring quantitative outcomes of care.

The reader can use the fundamental concepts and procedures presented here to launch a program of outcomes measurement. As the program expands, it will be helpful to use a statistical consultant for more advanced procedures and designs. In particular, cost analysis is a complex field, and a consultant can be essential in designing the collection and analysis of data on cost of care. Statistical consultation is most helpful during the initial design of the study and during data analysis and interpretation.

Although this chapter does not discuss the analysis of qualitative data, there are excellent texts and computer programs to guide the analysis of qualitative data. Certainly, qualitative data can be very informative in gaining a richer, more comprehensive understanding of patient outcomes of care. In addition, qualitative research can provide the basis for the development of new quantitative instruments.

MEASUREMENT CONCEPTS

Statistical procedures give organization and meaning to data. Statistics summarize data and readily identify outliers. In addition, statistics lend power to decision making by quantifying outcomes of care and answering research questions.

Level of Measurement

The first step in data analysis is to identify the level of measurement of the selected outcomes. The type of statistical procedure appropriate for evaluating patient outcomes or answering a research question depends on the level of measurement of the variables being examined. Generally, the higher the level of measurement, the greater flexibility available in choosing statistical procedures (Polit & Hungler, 1999). *Nominal* measurement (the lowest of the four levels) is used to classify attributes or objects into categories that are exclusive (e.g., gender, marital status, and medical diagnosis), with numbers assigned to represent categories of the attributes. Data analysis at this level is limited to descriptive statistics and commonly includes a frequency count of objects in each category and the percentage of the total. For example, the sample may consist of 50 subjects—41 (82%) married, 6 (12%) never married, and 3 (6%) divorced or widowed.

Data measured at the *ordinal* level can be assigned to categories that show relative rankings. The intervals between the rankings are not necessarily equal. Suppose educational level of subjects is categorized in the following groups: less than high school (coded as 1), high school diploma (coded as 2), baccalaureate degree (coded as 3), and graduate education (coded as 4). The amount of education can be ranked but graduate level (4) is not equal to twice as much education as high school (2). As another example of relative rankings, Likert-type attitudinal scales characterized by degrees of agreement with a statement (1 = strongly disagree, 2 = disagree, 3 = neutral, 4 = agree, and 5 = strongly agree) are very common in nursing research. Table 4.1 provides examples of variables at the nominal and ordinal levels.

Interval measurement shows rankings on a scale with equal intervals between the numbers. The zero point, however, remains arbitrary because there is no true zero point on the interval scale. Measurement of temperature on the Fahrenheit scale is a classic example of this level of measurement. Interval-level data permit greater statistical manipulation, such as calculation of mean scores.

Ratio measurement ranks variables on scales with equal intervals and absolute zeros. Examples of ratio-level data are intake and output, weight, pulse,

TABLE 4.1 Examples of Nominal- and Ordinal-Level Data

Variable	*Values*
Nominal level	
Gender	1 = Male
	2 = Female
Marital status	1 = Married
	2 = Never married
	3 = Divorced or widowed
Ordinal level	
Educational level	1 = Less than high school
	2 = High school graduate
	3 = College graduate
	4 = Graduate degree
Patient satisfaction scale	1 = Very dissatisfied
	2 = Somewhat dissatisfied
	3 = Neutral
	4 = Somewhat satisfied
	5 = Very satisfied

and length of stay (measured in days). All mathematical procedures can be performed on ratio-level data, and any statistical procedure is possible if appropriate.

STATISTICAL ANALYSES AND LEVEL OF MEASUREMENT

Differentiating between interval- and ratio-level data—that is, deciding whether a scale has a true zero—is sometimes a complex issue. In most cases, the differentiation is unnecessary because common statistical procedures can be performed on both levels of data.

Because the level of measurement of data determines the statistical analyses that can be performed, it is wise to obtain the highest level of measurement possible. For example, obtain patients' specific ages rather than collecting these data in ordinal categories of 20 to 29, 30 to 39, 40 to 49, and so on. This will permit calculation of a mean age for the sample and more sophisticated statistical procedures. The ages can be recoded easily into categories using SPSS should you decide to present the data by decades of age.

Nominal- and ordinal-level data are considered categorical and are appropriately analyzed using nonparametric statistical procedures. Interval- and ratio-level data are considered continuous and may be analyzed using more powerful parametric statistical procedures. Parametric procedures, however, must meet rigorous assumptions not required of nonparametric statistics. There is a controversy related to whether ordinal data used in psychosocial instruments such as Likert scales do not have an underlying interval continuum that justifies the use of parametric statistics (Waltz, Strickland, & Lenz, 1991). In fact, mean scores are commonly calculated for these instruments, and parametric procedures such as the *t* test are used to compare mean scores for two groups. This more liberal position is widely accepted in behavioral research. The Patient Satisfaction Scale in Table 4.1 is an example of an instrument that might be used in comparing two groups using the parametric statistic *t* test.

DATA ANALYSIS

There are three basic and logically progressive steps in data analysis: (a) describe the sample, (b) describe the scores on outcomes measures, and (c) test research hypotheses. The level of data analysis chosen depends on the nature of the patient outcomes project. Data analysis usually begins with a comprehensive description of the sample as the first step, including a description and comparison of specific groups within the sample. For example, in a study of patient satisfaction in the outpatient surgery setting, the first step involves describing the number of patients of each gender, the mean ages, the types of surgical procedures, and so on. Step two involves a description of the scores of the entire sample on the outcomes of interest, such as patient satisfaction, length of stay, cost of care, and quality of life. In this case, what is the current level of patient satisfaction in the outpatient surgery setting?

The final step of data analysis involves evaluating the effects of an intervention or testing other research hypotheses. For example, one might compare the satisfaction level of patients whose care is managed by advanced practice case managers to the satisfaction level of patients without case managers. It is helpful to develop a plan for data analysis similar to the one shown in Table 4.2.

Statistics are classified as either descriptive or inferential. Descriptive statistics, such as mean scores and percentages, describe and organize data. Inferential statistics are those used to make inferences or draw conclusions about a population from data collected on a sample drawn from that population.

TABLE 4.2 Plan for Data Analysis of Patient Satisfaction Data

Variable	Data Source	Level of Measurement	Statistical Procedure
Demographic			
Age	Medical record	Ratio	Mean, range
Gender	Medical record	Nominal	Frequency
Length of stay	Medical record	Ratio	Mean, *SD,* range, frequency, *t* test to compare groups
Satisfaction	Patient satisfaction	Ordinal (treated as interval)	Mean, *SD,* range, frequency, *t* test to compare groups

DESCRIPTIVE STATISTICS

A set of data can be described comprehensively by three characteristics: the shape of the distribution of values, the central tendency, and the variability.

Frequency Distributions

A frequency distribution is a systematic arrangement of data values from lowest to highest, with a count of the number of times each value occurred. Figure 4.1 shows a frequency distribution of ages of a sample of patients—first as individual scores in a bar chart and then as grouped according to decade in a histogram. Frequency data can be graphically displayed in bar, pie, and area charts and histograms as discussed in Chapter 5.

Measures of Central Tendency

Measures of central tendency give a single number that describes the distribution of values within the group or sample. Common measures of central tendency include the mode, the median, and the mean. The *mode* is the most frequent score and can be readily identified by inspection of an ungrouped frequency distribution of the data. A distribution of scores may be multimodal— that is, have more than one mode. The bar chart in Figure 4.1 provides an example of a multimodal distribution. The ages of 37 and 50 years each occur approximately 52 times. This is the highest frequency in the age distribution.

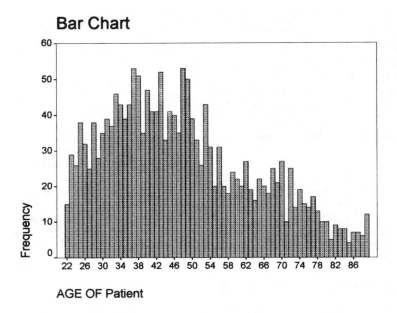

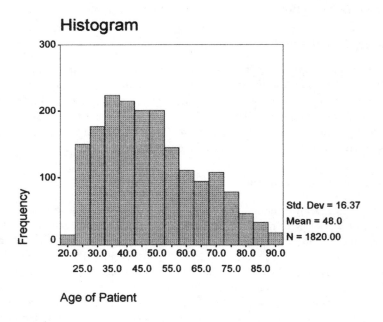

Figure 4.1. Frequency Distribution of Patient Age

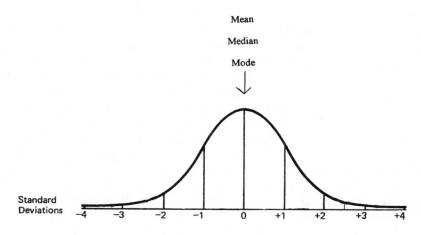

Figure 4.2. Normal Distribution With Standard Deviations

The *median* is the middle score and lies at the 50th percentile of the distribution of scores. If the number of scores is uneven, exactly 50% of the scores are higher than the median and 50% are lower (e.g., the 8th score in a set of 15 scores). If the number of scores is even, the median is the average of the two middle scores (e.g., 7.5 in a set of 14 scores when scores are "1 through 14"). The median is not sensitive to extreme scores and may best reflect the "typical" score when extreme scores skew the data.

The *mean* is the most commonly used and considered the most stable measure of central tendency. The mean represents the arithmetical average of all scores at interval- or ratio-level data and is calculated by summing all the scores and dividing by the number of scores in the set. Most tests of statistical significance use the group or sample mean score. If the distribution of scores is symmetrical and unimodal, the mean, median, and mode will coincide—as they do in the theoretical normal distribution shown in Figure 4.2.

Measures of Variability

Common measures of variability, such as the range of scores and the standard deviation, reflect the degree of homogeneity or heterogeneity of a sample. The range is the difference between the highest and the lowest scores and should always be accompanied by additional descriptive statistics. A sample with a wide range of ages of subjects, such as 10 to 78 years, is more heterogeneous (i.e., more variable) than a sample with a range of ages from 45 to 65 years.

The standard deviation is the most frequently used measure of variability with interval- or ratio-level data. The standard deviation reflects the average deviation of scores from the mean score. Both the sample with ages ranging from 10 to 75 years and the sample with ages ranging from 45 to 65 years may have a mean age of 52, but the standard deviation of the first sample will be larger than the standard deviation of the latter sample. The standard deviation is the square root of the variance, or variability of the scores.

When referring to critical pathways, the term *variance* is commonly used as a dichotomous variable (i.e., the patient met or did not meet a target along the pathway). Case managers sometimes add the number and causes of "variances" and design interventions based on this type of data to increase adherence to the pathway. We recognize the wide acceptability of this definition of variance and have even included such references in this book. We wish to gently persuade readers to use the term "pathway departure" to more accurately describe an unmet target on a critical pathway. Frequency analysis would be appropriate to summarize how many times a particular pathway departure occurred. Once the frequency of departures has been examined, however, it is important to examine the variability in the data. Knowing the extent to which the patients in a particular group deviated from the pathway can guide interventions in a more precise way. For example, Figure 13.2 in Chapter 13 displays the number of patients who regain continence during each week following prostatectomy. If Marschke had established Postoperative Week 17 as the target time by which patients would regain continence, she would have reported that 30 (88%) of the patients who achieved continence did so by the target date, with a pathway departure occurring in 4 (12%) patients. In fact, the mean time period at which continence was achieved was Postoperative Week 10, with a standard deviation of 6.7. This information indicates that an earlier target date for continence may be possible. The variability within this group, however, suggests that more than one type of intervention may be needed to assist patients to meet the target continence date. Patients who achieved continence by Week 12 may have simply needed more encouragement to perform exercises, whereas patients who did not achieve continence until after Week 15 may have needed a different type of exercise or additional medical intervention.

Bivariate Descriptive Statistics

For research concerned with relationships between variables, bivariate descriptive statistics are used. A contingency table is often used to display a two-dimensional frequency in which the frequencies of two variables measured at the nominal or ordinal level are cross-tabulated. Table 4.3 shows fictitious data for males and females on exercise behavior. Percentages are computed for the number of cases within each cell of the contingency table.

TABLE 4.3 Contingency Table for Gender and Exercise Behavior Relationship

Gender	Sedentary	Exercise Occasionally	Exercise Regularly	Total
		Exercise Behavior		
Male	60 (50% of males)	30 (25% of males)	30 (25% of males)	120 (55% of sample)
Female	65 (65% of females)	22 (22% of females)	13 (13% of females)	100 (45% of sample)
Total	125 (57% of sample)	52 (24% of sample)	43 (19% of sample)	220 (100% of sample)

Correlation procedures are also used to describe the relationship between two variables. A correlation coefficient from −1.00 to 1.00 can be calculated that describes the intensity and direction of variables measured at ordinal and higher levels. In a positive relationship, the higher the score on one variable, the higher the score on the other (e.g., pain and anxiety). In a negative or inverse relationship, higher scores on one variable are associated with lower scores on the other (e.g., pain and satisfaction with care). When variables are unrelated, the correlation coefficient is zero. A correlation of .80 is generally considered to represent a strong, positive relationship, whereas a correlation of −.20 represents a weak negative relationship (Munro, 1997). With unmanaged pain and anxiety, a correlation of .80 would indicate that higher levels of pain are associated with high levels of anxiety.

The product-moment correlation coefficient commonly referred to as Pearson's *r* is computed when variables are interval- or ratio-level data. The comparable correlation procedure for ordinal-level data is Spearman's rank-order correlation (r_s) or Spearman's rho. A two-dimensional correlation matrix displays the correlation of several variables to all the other variables in the matrix. Table 4.4 represents a correlation matrix from a study of factors related to fatigue in cancer patients receiving radiation therapy.

INFERENTIAL STATISTICS AND HYPOTHESIS TESTING

Outcomes research focuses on the outcomes of specific interventions for actual or potential health problems. This frequently involves comparison of outcomes

TABLE 4.4 Correlation Matrix: Symptoms of Cancer Patients Receiving Radiation Therapy[a]

	Fatigue	Anxiety	Depression	Insomnia
Fatigue	1.00			
Anxiety	0.60	1.00		
Depression	0.61	0.92	1.00	
Insomnia	0.55	0.59	0.52	1.00

a. All correlations significant at the .01 level.

from a group receiving a specific treatment to national norms, to a control group, or to a baseline measure of a variable of interest before the intervention was instituted. The strength of differences between groups is evaluated in terms of their statistical significance or the probability that the difference would have occurred by chance.

Inferential statistics are used to draw conclusions about a population on data drawn from a sample (e.g., in hypothesis testing). The researcher may be interested in determining the effectiveness of an intervention for all patients with chronic leg ulcers but tests the intervention on half of a sample of 100 patients with chronic leg ulcers treated at a specific medical center. The other half of the sample will be a control group receiving the usual care provided for such ulcers at that institution. The researcher's objective is to generalize the results from the research on 100 patients to all patients with similar leg ulcers. Statistical hypothesis testing provides objective criteria for making decisions about the outcome of the study. In this case, the research or *scientific hypothesis* is that there is a difference in group outcomes that is the result of the intervention being tested. The *null hypothesis,* which is the reverse hypothesis that is actually tested by statistical methods, in this case states that there is no difference between the groups that is not due to chance fluctuations.

Level of Significance

The level of significance or alpha level is the probability of rejecting a true null hypothesis. This is the same as deciding that a difference between groups exists (or a relationship between variables is present) when, in fact, it does not. This decision is also a Type I error. A Type II error is the decision that no difference exists between groups when, in fact, there is a true difference between groups (or a relationship between variables). In a Type II error, the null hypothesis was not rejected, although it should have been.

The minimum level of significance acceptable in scientific research is .05. This means that if a particular study were conducted 100 times on different samples of patients, a true null hypothesis would be rejected five times when it should not have been. In 95 of the samples, however, a true null hypothesis would be accepted as correct. When the level of significance is changed to a more conservative .01, the risk of a Type I error is lower and the null hypothesis will be erroneously rejected in only 1 sample in 100. The main reason not to consistently use an alpha level of .01 is that lowering the risk of making a Type I error increases the risk of making a Type II error. The stricter the criteria for rejecting a null hypothesis, the greater the risk of accepting a false null hypothesis that should be rejected. The .05 level of significance is considered by most researchers to be a reasonable balance between the two risks.

COMPARING GROUPS

The appropriate test statistic for comparing two or more groups or measuring pretest to posttest changes in a one-group sample is determined by the level of measurement of the dependent variable. The independent variable of "group" is measured at the nominal level (e.g., experimental vs. control, males vs. females, and freshman vs. sophomores vs. juniors vs. seniors). If the dependent variable is also measured at the nominal level, the appropriate test is the chi-square (χ^2) test. Chi-square is a nonparametric statistic used to determine whether the frequency in each category is different from what would be expected by chance. For example, a researcher may be evaluating a specific intervention to decrease falls in hospitalized elderly patients compared to a current fall-prevention protocol. The independent variable would be group: experimental (new intervention) versus control (current protocol). The dependent variable would be observed frequency of falls in each of the two groups. If there are fewer falls in the new intervention group, and if the calculated chi-square is large enough to be statistically significant, the researcher would conclude that the difference in frequency of falls in the two groups would not occur on the basis of chance alone and the null hypothesis (of no difference between groups) would be rejected. The researcher would also conclude that the new intervention is more effective in preventing falls than the current protocol (Figure 4.3). When sample sizes are small and expected frequencies are less than five in 20% of the cells, the Fisher's exact probability test is used.

When the dependent variable is measured at the ordinal level (e.g., functional status on a 5-point scale), the nonparametric statistical test of Mann-Whitney *U* is used to compare ranks of scores for two independent groups (the Kruskall-Wallis test is used for three or more groups). If a researcher is comparing baseline (or preintervention) scores to those of the same group after a specific intervention, the group scores are considered to be related or dependent rather

Group Patients Who Fell Crosstabulation

			Patients Who Fell		Total
			yes	no	
Group	Experimental	Count	30	510	540
		% within Group	5.6%	94.4%	100.0%
		% within Patients who Fell	42.9%	56.0%	55.1%
	Control	Count	40	400	440
		% within Group	9.1%	90.9%	100.0%
		% within Patients who Fell	57.1%	44.0%	44.9%
Total		Count	70	910	980
		% within Group	7.1%	92.9%	100.0%
		% within Patients who Fell	100.0%	100.0%	100.0%

Chi-Square Tests

	Value	df	Asymp. Sig. (2-sided)	Exact Sig. (2-sided)	Exact Sig. (1-sided)
Pearson Chi-Square	4.569[b]	1	.033		
Continuity Correction[a]	4.051	1	.044		
Likelihood Ratio	4.541	1	.033		
Fisher's Exact Test				.035	.022
Linear-by-Linear Association	4.564	1	.033		
N of Valid Cases	980				

a. Computed only for a 2 × 2 table.
b. 0 cells (.0%) have expected count less than 5. The minimum expected count is 31.43.

Figure 4.3. SPSS® Computer Printout: Chi-Square Analysis for Cross-Tabulation of Group by Patients Who Fell (Reproduced With Permission of SPSS, Inc.)

TABLE 4.5 Guide to Selecting Appropriate Statistical Tests

Parametric Tests (Test Statistic)	*Nonparametric Tests (Test Statistic)*
Difference between two independent groups	
t Test for independent groups (*t*)	Chi-square test (χ^2; difference in proportions, nominal data)
	Mann-Whitney *U* (*u*; ordinal data)
Difference between two sets of scores for the same group	
t Test for dependent groups (*t*)	McNemar's Chi-square test (χ^2; nominal data)
	Fisher's exact test when $N < 30$
	Wilcoxon signed-rank test (*z*; ordinal data)
Differences among three or more groups	
Analysis of variance (*F*)	Chi-square (χ^2; nominal data)
	Kruskall-Wallis (*H*; ordinal data)
Relationships between variables	
Pearson's *r*	Chi-square (χ^2; nominal data)
	Spearman's rank order correlation (r_s; ordinal data)

than independent, and a different statistical test is used (Wilcoxon signed-rank test). When the dependent variable is measured at the interval or ratio level (e.g., weight in kilograms), mean scores are calculated for the groups and the *t* test for independent samples is used to compare two groups. An analysis of variance (ANOVA) test would be used to compare the mean scores for three or more groups. Table 4.5 provides a brief guide to the selection of appropriate statistical tests for hypothesis testing.

ANALYZING DATA USING SPSS

Once patient outcomes data have been entered into an SPSS data file, SPSS can be used to describe the sample, examine relationships between variables, com-

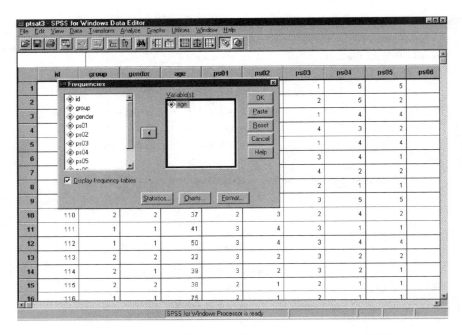

Figure 4.4. SPSS Data Analysis Procedure: Frequencies (Reproduced With Permission of SPSS, Inc.)

pare groups, or conduct whatever statistical analysis procedures are indicated to answer the research questions.

In the *Data Editor,* click on the word *Analyze* at the top of the page to open the data analysis menu. Note that this initial classification of analysis procedures includes *Descriptive Statistics* to describe data, *Compare Means* to conduct *t*-test group comparisons, *Correlate* to analyze the relationships between or among variables, *Nonparametric Tests* to carry out procedures using nonparametric tests such as Mann-Whitney *U,* and several other options for selected data analysis procedures.

Summarizing the Data

The *Frequencies* procedure is a good way to obtain basic descriptive statistics from your data and to search for errors in data entry. In the *Data Editor,* click on *Analyze* and move the cursor pointer to *Descriptive Statistics.* Next, click on *Frequencies,* and the *Frequencies* dialog box appears (Figure 4.4). From the

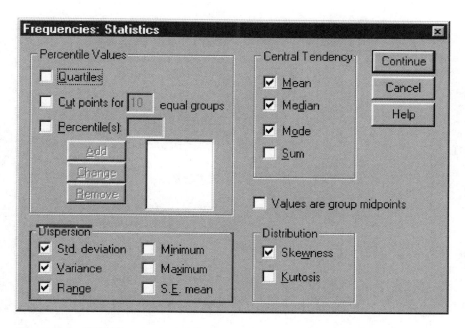

Figure 4.5. SPSS Data Analysis Procedure: Descriptive Statistics (Reproduced With Permission of SPSS, Inc.)

window in the left side of the box, select all variables that you would like described and move them into the window on the right by clicking the arrow between the windows. Next, click on the gray *Statistics* box at the bottom of the dialog box, and a variety of descriptive statistical procedures will appear. Select central tendency statistics, such as *Mean, Median,* and *Mode*; percentile values; measures of dispersion (variability), such as *Std. deviation* and *Range*; and statistics that describe the shape and symmetry of the distribution (Figure 4.5).

When appropriate statistics have been selected, click *Continue* to return to the *Frequencies* dialog box. Click on *Charts* to select *Bar Charts, Pie Charts, Histograms,* or no charts for display of the variables. Consult Chapter 5 for more detailed information on graphics using SPSS. Next, click on *Continue* to return to the dialog box, and then click on *Format.* Select the order in which you want results displayed (ascending vs. descending) and click on *Suppress tables with more than 10 categories* if you want to omit lengthy frequency displays such as the ages of 100 subjects. Click *Continue* to return to the dialog box, and click *OK* for the data analysis procedure to run. The results will be displayed in the *Output Viewer* window and may be printed or saved in a permanent file or both.

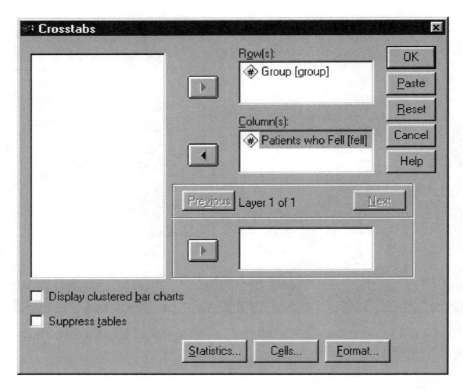

Figure 4.6. SPSS Data Analysis Procedure: Crosstabs (Reproduced With Permission of SPSS, Inc.)

Chi-Square

To perform a chi-square analysis, select *Analyze* and then *Descriptive Statistics* and then *Crosstabs* (Figure 4.6). From the variable box at the left, arrow over one variable into the box labeled *Row* and another variable into the box labeled *Column.* Then click the gray box labeled *Statistics* at the bottom of the dialog box. Click on *Chi square,* and then select *Continue.* Next, click on the gray box labeled *Cells* and select *Row* and *Column.* Next, click on *Continue,* and then click on *OK.* Figure 4.3 shows the results of a chi-square procedure comparing the proportion of patient falls under an experimental protocol to that of a control group. This figure reveals that 5.6% of patients in the experimental group fell, whereas 9.1% of patients in the control group fell. From the lower half of Figure 4.3, one can see that the Pearson Chi-square value for this analysis was 4.57 with a *p* value of .03. Because the *p* value is less than .05, this indicates that there is a significant difference in the fall rate for patients in the experimental group and patients in the control group.

Comparing Means (*t* Test)

For a *t* test comparison of group means, click on *Analyze* and then *Compare Means*. Select from the menu *Means* to compare means of a list of dependent variables within one or more independent variables, *One-Sample t* test to compare a group mean to a normative value, *Independent Sample t* test to compare means of two independent groups, *Paired-Samples t* test to compare paired scores within the same group as pretest to posttest scores, and *One-Way ANOVA* to compare means of three or more groups. For example, to compare the mean outpatient satisfaction scores of those receiving care by case managers versus those receiving usual care, click on *Independent Sample t Test* from the variable list on the left side of the dialog box, select *patient satisfaction total,* and move it to the window labeled *Test Variable(s)*. Click on *group* from the variable list, and move the variable under *Grouping Variable*. When *Define Groups* appears in the dialog box, enter "1" (defined as the group with case managers) for Group 1 and "2" (defined as "usual care") for Group 2 (Figure 4.7). Click on *Continue* to return to the original dialog box. Next, click *OK* to run the program. The output window will show both Levene's test for equality of variances and the *t* test for equality of means of the two groups (Figure 4.8). The *t* test requires that the two groups being compared have similar variances and the Levene's test indicates whether or not the groups have similar variances in total patient satisfaction scores. Because the *F* of the Levene's test is not significant (<.05), we conclude that the variances are equal and use the *t*-test statistic based on equal variances.

Reading from the *t* test result labeled "Equal Variances Assumed," it can be seen that the *t* value is 2.37 with a probability of .02. Because this is less than our selected alpha level of .05, we conclude that outpatient surgery patients whose care is managed by case managers are more satisfied with their care than patients in the standard care group.

Correlating Variables

To determine the correlation between patients' ages and their satisfaction scores, click on *Analyze* and then on *Correlate*. Select *Bivariate* because this is a correlation between two variables. In the dialog box, arrow the variables of *age* and *patient satisfaction total* (the Patient Satisfaction Scale total score) from the variable list on the left into the *Variable* box on the right (Figure 4.9). From the indicated options of correlations (*Pearson, Kendall's Tau-b,* or *Spearman*),

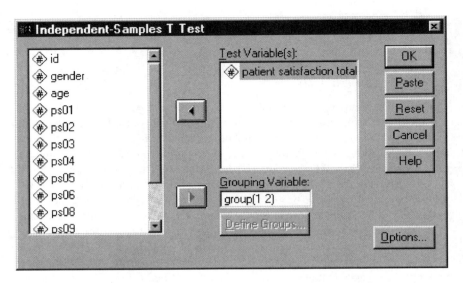

Figure 4.7. SPSS Data Analysis Procedure: *t* Test (Reproduced With Permission of SPSS, Inc.)

click on *Pearson.* Then, under *Test of Significance* select *Two-tailed* or *One-tailed* according to the study hypothesis. Click on *Flag significant correlations,* and then click on *OK* to run the analysis. Figure 4.10 shows the output, which shows a correlation of −.09, a weak inverse association between age and patient satisfaction with a *p* value of .52, indicating that the relationship between age and satisfaction was not a significant one in this study.

Checking the Reliability of Instruments

It is always a good idea to check the internal consistency reliability (Cronbach's alpha) of an instrument used in a particular sample of subjects. This process reveals to what extent the entire instrument is measuring the same construct. To do so, select *Analyze,* and then select *scale.* Next, select *Reliability Analysis.* Select and arrow over all the variables that represent scale items (or questions) from the box at the left into the white *Items* box at the right (Figure 4.11). In the white box labeled *Model,* click on *Alpha* (for Cronbach's alpha) from the selection of *Alpha, Split-half, Guttman,* and *Parallel.* Click on *Statistics* to select descriptive statistics, interitem correlations, and other statistics of interest. Next, click *Continue* and then *OK.* The resulting correlation of test items to total score indicates how well the individual questions measure similar concepts and how reliable the questionnaire was for testing of this sample.

Group Statistics

	Group Assignment	N	Mean	Std. Deviation	Std. Error Mean
Patient satisfaction total	1	24	35.96	8.04	1.64
	2	28	30.14	9.46	1.79

Independent Samples Test

		Levene's Test for Equality of Variances		t-test for Equality of Means					95% Confidence Interval of the Difference	
		F	Sig.	t	df	Sig. (2-tailed)	Mean Difference	Std. Error Difference	Lower	Upper
Patient satis-faction total	Equal variances assumed	1.487	.228	2.367	50	.022	5.82	2.46	.88	10.75
	Equal variances not assumed			2.397	49.998	.020	5.82	2.43	.94	10.69

Figure 4.8. SPSS® Computer Printout: *t* Test for Independent Samples (Reproduced With Permission of SPSS, Inc.)

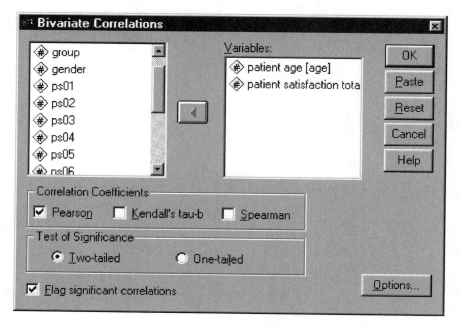

Figure 4.9. SPSS Data Analysis Procedure: Pearson's Correlation (Reproduced With Permission of SPSS, Inc.)

INTERPRETATION OF FINDINGS

The interpretation of study results involves a determination of the accuracy of the findings, their meaning and importance, their generalization, and their implications.

Assessment of the accuracy of study findings requires a review of the study methods and the extent to which extraneous variables were controlled. Study limitations should be identified and discussed. In addition, if the null hypothesis could not be rejected, a power analysis (with the help of a statistical consultant) can determine the likelihood that a Type II error occurred because the sample size was too small. Finally, an evaluation of the instruments used to measure outcomes may reveal deficits in performance that undermine the determination of intervention effectiveness.

The meaning and importance of the findings should be evaluated both statistically and clinically. Nonsignificant statistical test results can have important clinical significance, such as a finding of no difference in the rate of complications for an "early discharge" group compared to a "usual length of stay" group.

Correlations

		Patient Age	Patient Satisfaction Total
Patient age	Pearson Correlation	1.000	-.092
	Sig. (2-tailed)		.515
	N	52	52
Patient satisfaction total	Pearson Correlation	-.092	1.000
	Sig. (2-tailed)	.515	
	N	52	52

Figure 4.10. SPSS Computer Printout: Correlation Between Age and Satisfaction Scores (Reproduced With Permission of SPSS, Inc.)

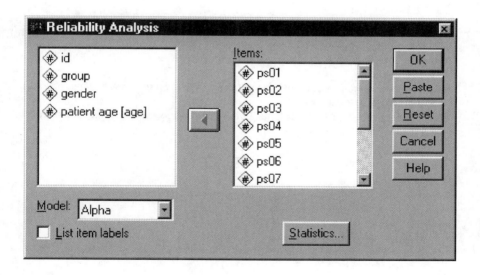

Figure 4.11. SPSS Data Analysis Procedure: Reliability Analysis (Reproduced With Permission of SPSS, Inc.)

A correlation of .15 between length of stay and patient satisfaction, however, may be statistically significant in a large sample but does not reflect a strong nor an important relationship between the two variables.

The aim of research is to be able to generalize results from the sample of subjects studied to the larger population of people with the particular problem under investigation. This requires a careful assessment of the extent to which the sample is similar to, and different from, the target population.

Interpretation of findings also includes implications of the results for clinical practice, for future research, for professional education, for development of theory, and for changes in health policy. Study findings should be compared to those of other researchers in the field and to the theoretical framework on which the study was based so that knowledge of the problem being studied can progress (Burns & Grove, 1997).

The research team should carefully identify the implications for clinical practice and for the development of health policy. Finally, the results should be shared with other professionals (and, if appropriate, with the public) so that patients and care providers in other settings can benefit from the research.

REFERENCES

Burns, N., & Grove, S. (1997). *The practice of nursing research: Conduct, critique, & utilization* (3rd ed.). Philadelphia: Saunders.
Munro, B. F. (1997). *Statistical methods for health care research* (3rd ed.). Philadelphia: J. B. Lippincott.
Polit, D. F., & Hungler, B. P. (1999). *Nursing research: Principles and methods* (6th ed.). Philadelphia: J. B. Lippincott.
Waltz, C. F., Strickland, O. L., & Lenz, E. R. (1991). *Measurement in nursing research* (2nd ed.). Philadelphia: Davis.

CHAPTER 5

Persuasive Presentation of Patient Outcomes Graphics

Marie T. Nolan

Knowing how to present patient data graphically can place nurses in a powerful position within institutions committed to achieving the best possible patient outcomes. Patient outcomes graphics can quickly summarize large amounts of data and help to guide the action of multidisciplinary groups charged with providing state-of-the-art care in a cost-effective manner. Examples of graphics that command attention are a line chart showing decreasing postoperative infection rates, a pie chart breaking down costs of care, and a box plot showing the variance in length of stay for patients on a critical pathway. Outcomes graphics can also be presented to payers who evaluate the quality and cost of care at several institutions before selecting a provider. Creating persuasive graphics requires selecting the appropriate graphic for the data; attending to details such as scale, color, and labeling; and tailoring the overall presentation to the interest of the audience. Learning these strategies will improve the reader's data presentation skills and ability to interpret and evaluate data graphics presented by others.

SELECTING THE APPROPRIATE GRAPHIC FOR THE DATA

Data may be presented in three ways: in the text of a report, in a table, or in a graphic (Tufte, 1983). One or two figures may easily be incorporated into a

TABLE 5.1 Demographic Data ($N = 96$)

Variable	Frequency	%
Gender		
Male	72	75
Female	24	25
Age		
40 to 65	29	30
65 and older	67	70
Admission status		
Emergency	2	2
Scheduled	70	73
Urgent	24	25
Surgical procedure		
Bypass	58	60
Bypass and valve	38	40

written report without interrupting its flow. Data involving multiple figures or many variables, however, may be most clearly presented in table format (Table 5.1). Other types of patient outcomes data, including the frequency and distribution of outcomes, relationships among outcomes, and changes in outcomes over time, can most effectively be presented in a graphic.

Frequency Data

Whether developing a critical pathway, evaluating its effect, or conducting a performance improvement project, frequency data are often the starting point for influencing patient outcomes. How many patients with a particular problem were treated, and what were their ages? What procedures did they undergo, and how many departments were involved in their care? These and similar questions are all answered with frequency data. Bar, pie, and area charts can be used to graphically present frequency data.

Variance Data

Many institutions, including some described in this book, refer to variance as a patient's departure from a target on a critical pathway. For example, using a

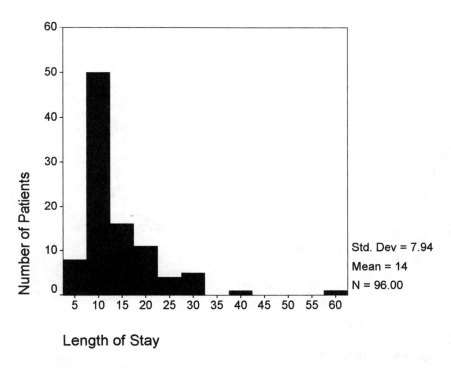

Figure 5.1. Length of Stay: Gastrointestinal Surgery

critical pathway for gastrointestinal surgery that has a length of stay of 7 days as the target, a stay longer than 7 days would be considered a variance. Efforts are then focused on identifying the reason for each variance and designing interventions to eliminate the variances. Additional analysis is required, however, to develop interventions specific enough to improve the care of patients who stay 8 days versus patients who stay from 30 to 60 days. In addition to tracking the number of pathway departures, outcomes managers need to also examine the spread or distribution of the data when planning improvements in care. The variance of a data set is a measure of dispersion around the mean that is equal to the square of the standard deviation. A large variance means that the data are widely distributed. Histograms offer a straightforward visual way of displaying the distribution of the data. The team working on improving the care of patients undergoing gastrointestinal surgery could begin to examine the data by creating a histogram of the length of stay (Figure 5.1).

Figure 5.1 immediately conveys the range in length of stay and where most patients fall on this continuum. The team can then decide to focus their efforts

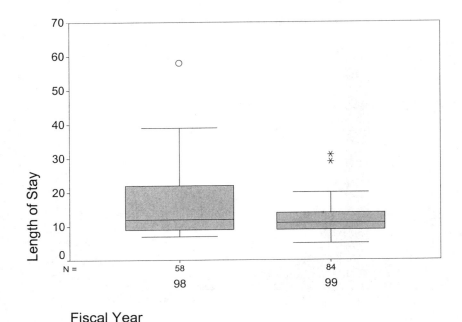

Figure 5.2. Length of Stay for Knee Replacement

on patients who stay just a few days beyond the target length of stay or on patients who stay 20 or more days longer than the target length of stay. Figure 5.1 reveals that most patients are hospitalized approximately 10 days. Only a few patients stay 15 days or longer. Improving care by early extubation after surgery or intensive care unit discharge on weekends may be needed to decrease the length of stay for patients in the 10-day group, whereas prevention of postoperative infections, ileus, or falls may be needed to decrease the length of stay for patients who stay longer than 15 days. Perhaps the senior clinicians on the surgical unit could improve the processes of care for patients in the 10-day group, whereas case managers or clinical nurse specialists may be required to manage the more complex care of patients in the >15-day group.

Boxplots are another excellent way to display the distribution of data for a particular variable for more than one patient group at a time. For example, Figure 5.2 shows the distribution in length of stay for patients undergoing knee surgery from one year to another.

The box in Figure 5.2 represents values from the 25th to the 75th percentile of the distribution. The dark horizontal line inside the box represents the median

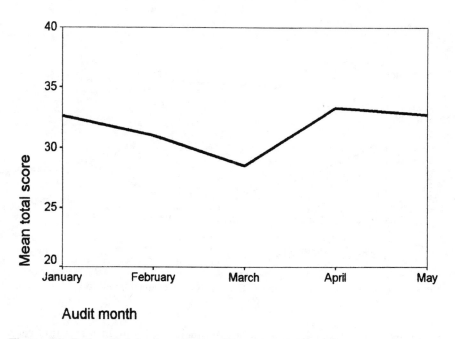

Audit month

Figure 5.3. Patient Satisfaction—January Through May ($N = 349$)

value, and the lines at the end of the boxes represent the largest and smallest values in the distribution that are not outliers. Open circles outside the lines represent outliers that are one and one-half to three box lengths from either end of the box. The star symbols outside the lines represents an extreme outlier that is more than three box lengths from either end of the box. Figure 5.2 shows that in 1999 patients undergoing knee replacement had a smaller distribution in length of stay and a shorter median length of stay than did patients in 1998. Like the histogram, the boxplot clearly identifies outliers and can therefore help to tailor performance improvement efforts for this group.

Time Series Data

Line charts can visually tell the story of changes in patient outcomes over time. Figure 5.3 reveals the average patient score on a satisfaction survey for five consecutive months.

This simple line chart easily draws the viewers' attention to the slight decrease in satisfaction during March. This is an excellent starting point for

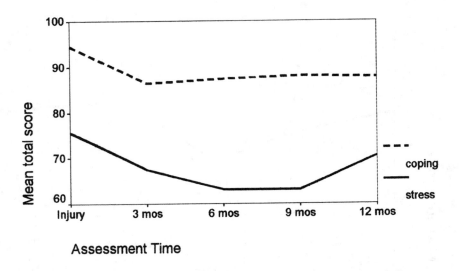

Figure 5.4. Family Stress and Coping Following Head Injury ($N = 245$)

examining patient satisfaction and all the factors that might affect this very important patient outcome.

Correlational Data

Multiple line charts and scatterplots can be used to illustrate the relationship between two variables. For example, the line chart in Figure 5.4 shows the relationship between stress level and coping efforts in families following the head injury of a family member.

The lines in Figure 5.4 represent mean stress and mean coping scores at several points in time. Clearly, the time of injury is the period of greatest stress. Although discharge planning now commonly begins at admission, Figure 5.4 helps one understand why family readiness to participate in these plans may be limited early in the injury period.

Scatterplots are unique because they reveal a relationship between two variables by showing each patient's score in a distribution. For example, nurses and physicians commonly assume that there is a strong relationship between patient age and length of stay. Patients older than 80 years of age might be predicted to have significantly longer stays than younger patients. If this were true, a scatterplot would show that as a patient's age increased so would the patient's length of stay. A scatterplot of age and length of stay for patients undergoing

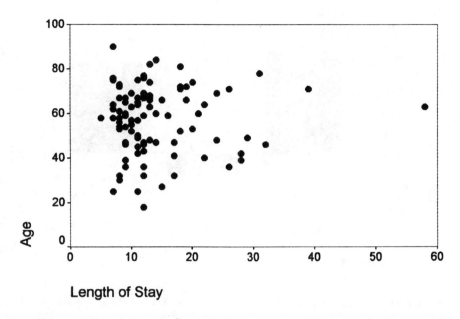

Figure 5.5. Length of Stay by Age (*N* = 96)

cardiac surgery, however, shows that the length of stay for patients 80 years old and older is very similar to that of patients in their 50s and 60s (Figure 5.5).

The patient with the longest length of stay in this distribution (58 days) is 63 years old. In this group of patients, there is no significant relationship between age and length of stay.

Benchmark Data

It is no longer sufficient for institutions to provide better care at a lower cost than they provided in previous years. Institutions must benchmark their patient outcomes against "best practice" outcomes. The hanging bar chart is a way to show the extent of deviation from the ideal. For example, River Hill Hospital is the hospital in a given health system that provides cardiac surgery for the lowest cost with outcomes similar to those at Exlenta, Hudson, and County Hospitals. Using River Hill Hospital as the benchmark institution, case managers begin to break down the costs of care for cardiac surgery patients and discover that the mean total laboratory charges at River Hill are $1,800. Figure 5.6 displays the $1,800 mean laboratory charge from River Hill as a line and the mean laboratory charges of the other hospitals as bars.

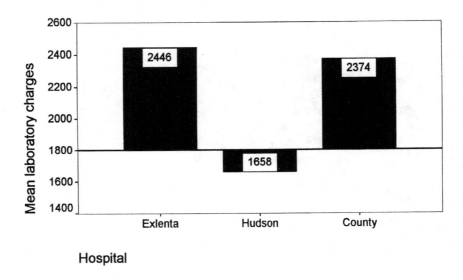

Figure 5.6. Mean Laboratory Charges for Diagnostic-Related Group 191 Compared to Those for River Hill Hospital (for Which Mean Laboratory Charges = $1,800)

The viewer can quickly see that although the mean laboratory charges of Hudson Hospital are lower than those of River Hill Hospital, the laboratory charges of Exlenta and County Hospitals are higher than those of River Hill Hospital. River Hill Hospital may be charged less by its laboratory or may have a more efficient system for communicating laboratory findings from the out-patient to the inpatient setting, thus eliminating the need for repeating blood tests unnecessarily. In any case, this graphic can serve to begin the analysis of this cost factor.

ATTENDING TO GRAPHIC DETAILS

Graphic Labels

The title of a graphic should identify the type of data presented, the total number of patients depicted, and the time period the data represent. A pie chart can be deceiving if it is unclear what the whole pie represents. For example, Figure 5.7 details the reasons for unplanned hospital admissions required by

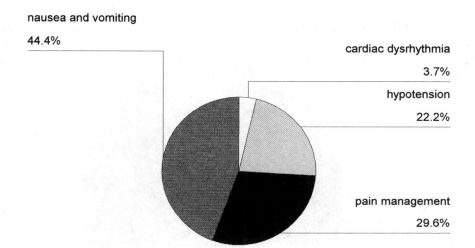

Figure 5.7. Reasons for Unplanned Admission Following Outpatient Knee Surgery (*N* = 3,255 Procedures)

1.4% of all patients undergoing outpatient knee surgery. The whole that the pie represents is only the 1.4% of patients with unplanned admissions.

Because the pie slices are identified by percentages, and the chart title identifies only the total number of patients undergoing knee surgery, one might assume that all patients who undergo knee surgery at this institution experience an unplanned hospital admission. Including the number of unplanned admissions next to the total number of admissions in the title would improve this chart. Alternately, preceding this chart with a pie chart that represents the total number of patients undergoing knee surgery, broken down into patients requiring and those not requiring unplanned admissions would clarify the data (Figure 5.8).

Graphic Order and Attributes

Presenting data chronologically or in ascending or descending order can make it easier to read than data that is randomly ordered. Also, value labels placed directly on a graph rather than alongside it can simplify the overall appearance of a graph and promote ease of interpretation. Although computerized graphics packages offer many options, such as color, shading, patterns, and

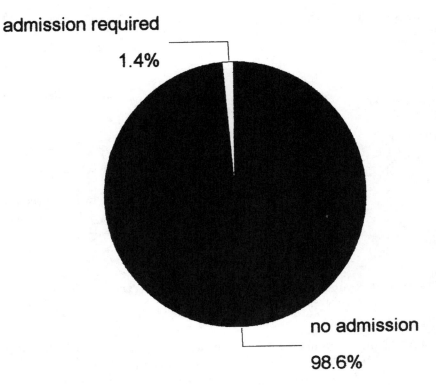

Figure 5.8. Frequency of Unplanned Admission Following Outpatient Knee Surgery
($N = 3,255$ Procedures)

three-dimensional effects, overuse of these attributes can detract from rather
than add to a graphic's message. Figure 5.9 is an overaccessorized graphic with
no meaningful order to its data.

Figure 5.10 represents the same data as that shown in Figure 5.9, only they are
presented in descending order with simplified features. The viewer need only
scan this graph once from left to right to know what percentage of hip replacements each payer accounts for and in what order.

Manipulating the scale used in a graphic can create a very different impres-
sion. Figure 5.11, which depicts 5-day survival rates following cardiac surgery
at four hospitals, uses the same data as those in Figure 5.12. In Figure 5.12, however, the survival rate scale ranges from 90% to 100% rather than from 98.5% to
99.2%, the scale range used in Figure 5.11.

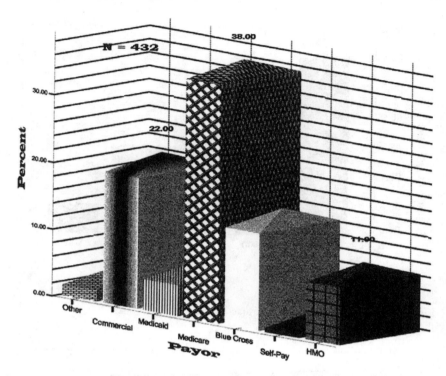

Figure 5.9. Percentage of Hip Replacements by Payor in Fiscal Year 1998

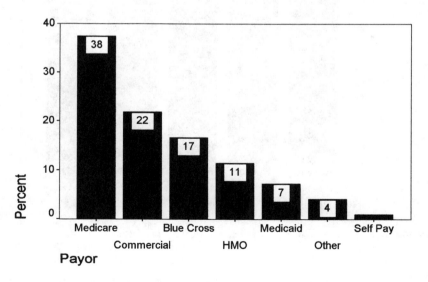

Figure 5.10. Percentage of Hip Replacements by Payor (N = 432)

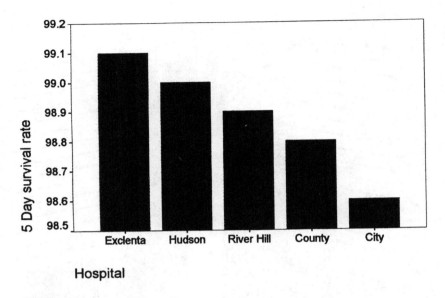

Figure 5.11. Metropolitan Area Cardiac Surgery Survival Rates

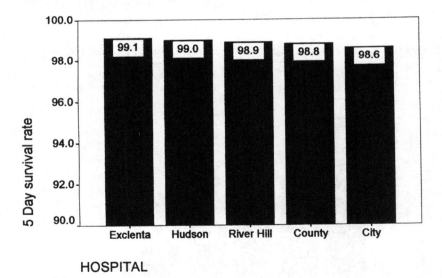

Figure 5.12. Metropolitan Area Cardiac Surgical Survival Rates

The change in scale makes the differences among the hospitals seem much greater than they are in reality. After all, the 0.5% difference in survival between Exclenta and City Hospitals could be due to chance rather than a true difference in quality of care. It is also unclear from the charts in Figures 5.11 and 5.12 how many patients these bars represent and what time period the data represent. Figure 5.11 should make the viewer suspect that this graphic was intended as an advertisement for Exclenta Hospital rather than as a straightforward treatment of patient outcomes data.

KNOWING THE TARGET AUDIENCE

Presenting data persuasively involves tailoring the presentation to meet the needs of the audience. A multidisciplinary committee working to streamline the care of the patient undergoing cardiac valve surgery may spend hours pouring over information about patient risk factors, cost of supplies and equipment, time to extubation after surgery, length of stay, and readmission rates. A payer negotiating a contract for cardiac care with this institution, however, may be interested only in data on cost of care and long-term survival rates. Jargon and abbreviations should be avoided if possible or defined in a graphic footnote or key.

WORKING WITH GRAPHICS
SOFTWARE PACKAGES

Charts or tables created from a statistical package such as SPSS (1998) can stand alone or be copied directly into the file of a graphics software program, such as Powerpoint (1997) or Harvard Graphics (1995). This allows the presenter to incorporate outcomes data into a presentation that includes slides that discuss the data and recommend action. Also, graphics programs have the flexibility to print out two to six slides per page if the presenter wishes to give the listeners a handout including several of the patient outcomes graphics. Printing multiple graphics on the same page can demonstrate the progression in the analysis of patient outcomes data from the general to the specific or from the past to the present.

Computer graphics programs also offer a wider range of options than most statistical packages in terms of background colors and designs. These options should be used with restraint, however, because too many bright colors and patterns in the background can detract from rather than emphasize the data (Wilkinson, 1994). Color within the graphic should call attention to the presenter's main point. For example, a presenter who wishes to have viewers focus on 5% of patients depicted in a pie chart who are in the highest severity of illness category could color this 5% pie slice red while using gray tones to depict patients in the other severity of illness categories. Simple contrasts may make a point more clearly than a rainbow of colors.

CREATING PATIENT OUTCOMES GRAPHICS USING SPSS

Once patient outcomes data are in an SPSS data file, SPSS can summarize these data by creating graphs and charts such as those presented in this chapter. For more advanced users of SPSS, there is an "interactive graphics" capability for many types of charts that allows for greater interaction between the database and the chart output. This introductory chapter on outcomes graphics, however, will describe the standard graphic commands of SPSS (1999).

Bar Charts

In the *Data Editor,* click the word *Graphs* at the top of the page to open the *Graphs* menu. Then click *Bar* to open the *Bar Charts* dialog box shown in Figure 5.13.

To create a simple bar chart in which the bars represent the number of persons of each gender, select the options for *Simple* and *Summaries for groups of cases.* Then click *Define.* In the *Define Simple Bar* dialog box, click the variable *gender* from the variable list. This activates the arrow next to the empty *Category Axis* box. Click once on this arrow to move the variable *gender* into the *Category Axis* box and notice that doing this causes the *OK* button to activate (Figure 5.14). Clicking the *OK* button will produce the viewer with the bar chart for gender on the right side of the screen and the output outline on the left side of the screen (Figure 5.15).

Each new chart created from the *Data Editor* will be deposited in the same viewer. The output outline provides an easy way to change the order of graphics in viewer. For example, to move a chart from the beginning to the end, click on the chart name at the beginning of the output outline and, while holding the left mouse button down, drag the chart icon to the end of the outline and release. The chart will then be at the end of the charts in the *Viewer.* The contents of the viewer can be saved at any time in an output file simply by clicking on *File* and *Save.* This type of file has an extension, *SPO.* Therefore, an output file made up of several graphics representing demographic data could be saved as *demographics.spo.*

To modify a chart—for example, by labeling the bars and adding a chart title—double click directly on the bar chart. This will produce the chart editor

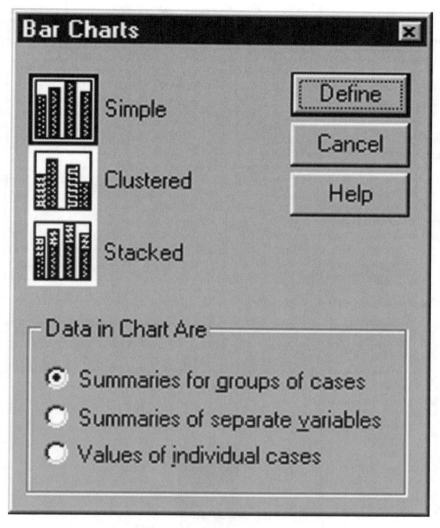

Figure 5.13. *Bar Charts* Dialog Box (Reproduced With Permission of SPSS, Inc.)

window. To label the bars, click *Format* and then *Bar Label Styles*. Click the picture of the labeling style desired, and then click *Apply All* and then click *Close*. While still in the chart editor window, click *Chart* and then *Title*. Enter a title in the *Title1* box and click *OK*.

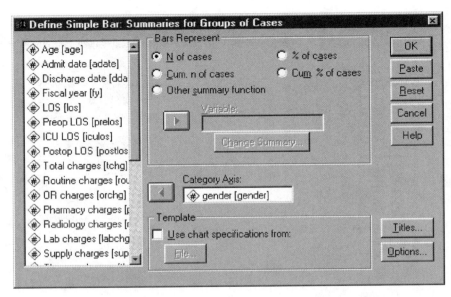

Figure 5.14. *Define Simple Bar* Dialog Box (Reproduced With Permission of SPSS, Inc.)

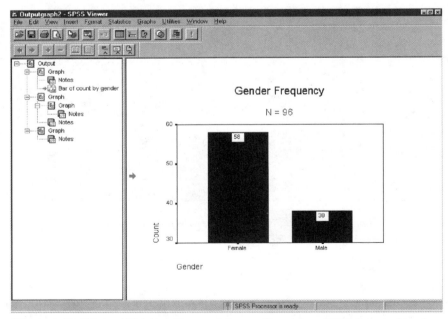

Figure 5.15. Viewer With Bar Chart and Output (Reproduced With Permission of SPSS, Inc.)

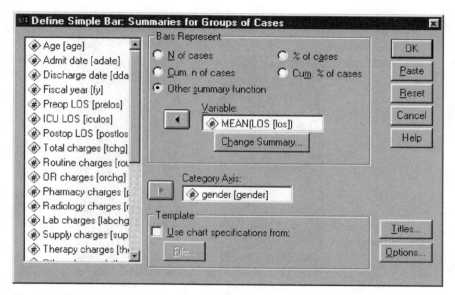

Figure 5.16. *Define Simple Bar* Dialog Box (Reproduced With Permission of SPSS, Inc.)

Bar charts can also represent values other than frequencies and can contain more than one variable. For example, to create a bar chart in which the bars represent the mean length of stay for males and females, from the *Data Editor* click on the word *Graphs* at the top of the page to open the *Graphs* menu. Then click *Bar* to open the *Bar Charts* dialog box shown in Figure 5.13. Select the options for *Simple* and *Summaries for groups of cases*. Then click *Define*. In the *Define Simple Bar* dialog box, click the variable *gender* from the variable list. This activates the arrow next to the empty *Category Axis* box. Click once on this arrow to move the variable *gender* into the *Category Axis* box. In the *Bars Represent* box, click on *Other summary function* and then click on the variable *LOS* to highlight it. Move the variable *LOS* into the variable box by clicking on the arrow next to this box. Notice that the word *mean* automatically appears by the variable label *LOS* in the variable box (Figure 5.16).

Click *OK* to produce the chart in the viewer. As before, double clicking directly on the bar chart will produce the chart editor, in which the chart title and bar labels can be added to produce the completed chart. Once the editing of the chart has been completed, close the chart editor by clicking on the *X* in the gray box in the upper right-hand corner of the screen. This will return you to the viewer. To print the chart from the viewer, click once on the chart to select

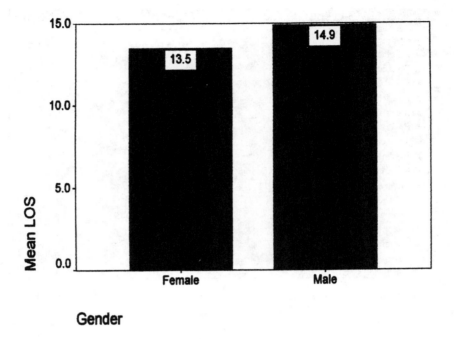

Figure 5.17. Mean Length of Stay by Gender ($N = 96$)

it for printing. Next, you can either click on the printer icon at the top of your screen or click on the word *File* at the top of the screen and then select *print* from the file menu. This will allow you to print out the graph you have selected from the viewer (Figure 5.17).

If you do not select a particular graph in the viewer to print out by clicking on it, all the graphs and analyses in the viewer will be printed out when you select the print command.

To create a bar chart that benchmarks a selected variable against a best prac-tice value as in Figure 5.6, first create a chart with the bars representing mean values as discussed previously. From the chart editor, double click on the left vertical axis scale to produce the *Scale Axis* dialog box. Click on the empty box labeled *Bar origin line* and enter the best practice value in the empty box at the right. In Figure 5.6, this would be the laboratory charge of $1,800. Then click *OK* to produce the final chart.

More complex bar charts can include more than two variables using clustered or stacked bars. A chart that displays the mean charges for laboratory, radiology,

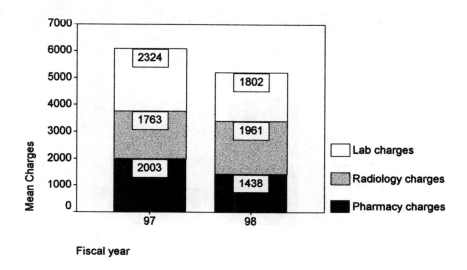

Figure 5.18. Breakdown of Mean Charges for Patients Undergoing Knee Replacement ($N = 540$)

and pharmacy services for fiscal years 1997 and 1998 is an example of a complex but extremely valuable graphic. To create this chart, from the *Graphs* menu click *Bar,* then *Stacked,* then *Summaries of separate variables,* and then click *Define.* In the *Define Stacked Bar* dialog box, highlight the variable *fiscal year* and move it into the *Category Axis* box by clicking the arrow next to this box. Next, highlight the variables *lab, radiology, and pharmacy,* and move them into the *Bars Represent* box by clicking the arrow next to this box. Notice that the word *mean* appears automatically next to the names of the three variables. Finally, click *OK* to produce the stacked bar chart in Figure 5.18.

Pie Charts

The commands for producing pie charts are very similar to those required for producing bar charts. From the *Data Editor,* click on *Graph,* then *Pie,,* then *Summaries for groups of cases,* and then *Define.* In the *Define pie* dialog box, select a variable from the list at the left to arrow into the *Define Slices by* box.

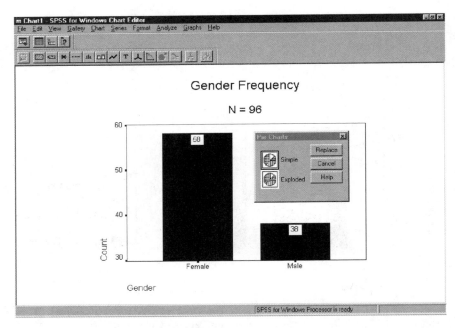

Figure 5.19. *Pie Charts* Dialog Box to Convert Bar Chart to Pie Chart (Reproduced With Permission of SPSS, Inc.)

In the *Slices Represent* box above, click on *N of cases* or one of the other summary functions, and then click *OK* to produce the chart.

Pie charts may also be created directly from bar charts. For example, double clicking on the bar chart in Figure 5.14 will produce the chart editor dialog box. From this dialog box, select *Gallery* and then *Pie* to produce the *Pie Charts* dialog box (Figure 5.19).

Next, click on the figure for a *simple* or *exploded* pie. Then click *Replace* to produce a pie chart in the viewer, and then select the pie chart and print it (Figure 5.20).

Histograms

Creating a histogram is very similar to creating a bar chart. In the *Data Editor,* click *Graphs* and then *Histogram.* From the *Histogram* dialog box, highlight the desired variable and click the arrow to move the variable into the *Variable* box. Finally, click *OK* to produce the chart.

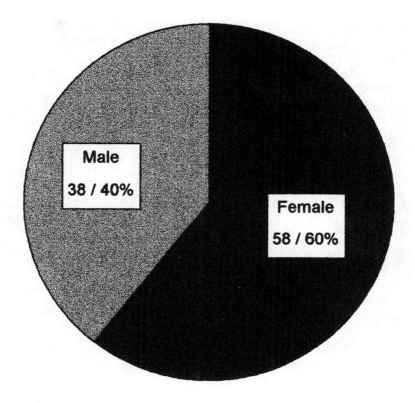

Figure 5.20. Gender Frequency (*N* = 96)

Line Charts

Creating line charts is very similar to creating bar charts. For example, to create a line chart similar to Figure 5.3, from the *Graphs* menu click *Line,* and from the *Line Charts* dialog box select *Simple* and *Summaries for groups of cases* and then click *Define* (Figure 5.21).

In the *Define Simple Line* dialog box, highlight the variable *audit month* and click the arrow next to the *Category Axis* box to move it into this box. Next, click on *Other summary function* and then highlight the variable *satisfaction sum* and move this variable into the *Variable* box by clicking the arrow next to this box. Finally, click *OK* to produce the chart in the viewer and then print the figure (Figure 5.22).

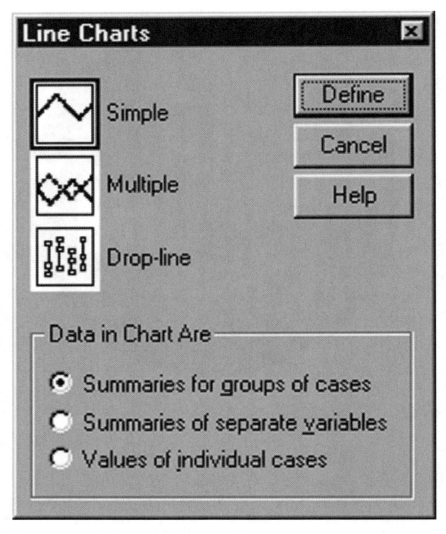

Figure 5.21. *Line Charts* Dialog Box (Reproduced With Permission of SPSS, Inc.)

Boxplots

To create a boxplot similar to Figure 5.2, from the *Graphs* menu click *Boxplot.* In the *Boxplot* dialog box, click *Simple* and *Summaries for groups of cases* and then *Define.* In the *Define Simple Boxplot* dialog box, highlight the

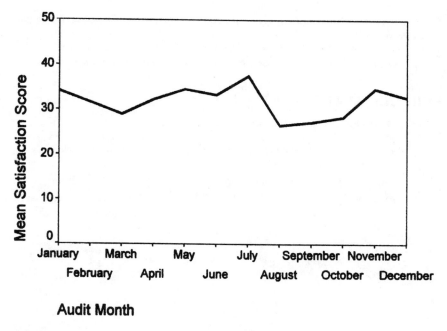

Audit Month

Figure 5.22. Mean Patient Satisfaction for 7 South (*N* = 120)

variable *LOS* and click the arrow to move *LOS* into the *Variable* box. Next, high-light the variable *fiscal year* and click the arrow to move it into the *Category Axis* box. Finally, click *OK* to create the boxplot.

SUMMARY

Obtaining and analyzing clinical data is only the first step in improving patient outcomes. Using graphics to persuasively present data can place nurses in a leadership position in the ongoing management of these outcomes.

REFERENCES

Harvard graphics Version 4 [Computer software]. (1995). Santa Clara, CA: Software Publishing.
Powerpoint Version 4 [Computer software]. (1997). Redmond, WA: Microsoft.
SPSS Version 9.0 [Computer software]. (1998). Chicago: SPSS.
SPSS. (1999). *SPSS base 9.0 applications guide.* Chicago: Author.

Tufte, E. R. (1983). *The visual display of quantitative information*. Cheshire, CT: Graphics Press.

Wilkinson, L. (1994). Less is more: Two- and three-dimensional graphics for data display. *Behavior Research Methods, Instruments, & Computers, 26*, 172-176.

FURTHER READING

Briscoe, M. (1996). *Preparing scientific illustrations* (2nd ed.). New York: Springer-Verlag.

McKinney, V., & Burns, N. (1993). The effective presentation of graphs. *Nursing Research, 42*, 250-252.

Wallgren, A., Wallgren, B., Persson, R., Jorner, U., & Haaland, J. (1996). *Graphing statistics & data, creating better charts*. Thousand Oaks, CA: Sage.

CHAPTER 6

Scanning Technology to Automate Data Entry

Laura J. Burke

Barbara F. Paegelow

"We are drowning in data, yet lack information!" This cry is often heard from clinical outcomes managers who face daily data management challenges. Use of scanning technology can help outcomes managers turn data into information by improving staff productivity and accuracy during the data entry process. In fact, Smyth, McIlvenny, Barr, Dickson, and Thompson (1997) found that optical scanning use for clinical data entry increased staff productivity sevenfold and decreased error rates from 12.4 errors per 1,000 responses for manual data entry to <0.2 errors per 1,000 responses for automated data. A variety of software programs exist to support clinical data management. Several of these programs are described in the literature cited under Further Reading. These programs range in price from $800 to approximately $2,000 and can be used in conjunction with a variety of scanners that range in price from a few hundred dollars to several thousand dollars.

AUTHORS' NOTE: We acknowledge the Outcomes Management Chartered Team, the Patient Pathway Process Team, the Variance Tracking Work Group, and the various patient pathway teams for their contribution to the development and maintenance of the Outcomes Variance Tracking Process in use at St. Luke's Medical Center, Milwaukee, Wisconsin. We also thank Lee Jeske, RN, BSN, Dona Hutson, RN, BSN, Marita Schifalacqua, RN, MSN, and Cindy Lewis, RN, MSN, for their thoughtful critique of the manuscript; Vicki George, RN, MSN, for her administrative support; and Kristin Baird for her technical expertise in manuscript preparation.

Since 1996, at St. Luke's Medical Center (Milwaukee, WI) we have used a low-cost combination of a Hewlett-Packard ScanJet IV scanner with a 50-page document feeder, a Pentium personal computer, Teleform Standard Version 5.3 software (1997), and a Hewlett-Packard LaserJet IV printer to create an outcomes variance tracking data entry system. The 1996 cost to purchase this system was slightly more than $4,000.

As director of nursing research and as the clinical information specialist, we served as leaders in introducing scanning technology for variance tracking. In this chapter, we will describe how the Teleform software works and how we developed and now maintain our variance tracking system. We hope that sharing this information will enable other organizations to develop similar variance tracking systems to support their outcomes management programs until outcome data are retrievable from automated patient records. Throughout the chapter, we use examples of our forms associated with various pathways to illustrate key concepts.

OVERVIEW OF TELEFORM
STANDARD VERSION 5.3

Teleform Standard Version 5.3 is a comprehensive software application that has three components: *Designer, Reader,* and *Verifier.* In *Designer,* a secretary with basic computer skills can create data collection forms and the forms' associated "code books" once the basic form has been drafted by someone experienced in instrument development. A variety of fonts, shapes, text, drawings, and data entry field choices are available for use to create the forms. These forms can be printed on letter- or legal-sized paper, can be single or multipaged, and can be distributed either by fax machine or in paper form.

To scan the data from a completed form into the form's database, the host computer must be powered on with the *Reader* program running. Data can be entered using one of two methods: through an optical scanner that is connected to the computer or through a fax machine that is connected to the computer via a modem phone line. Scanning tends to be most users' favored mode of data entry because it is faster, easier, and can be supervised by someone with minimal training. Faxed data input, however, is also a desirable option because forms can be faxed in at anytime from anywhere.

The *Verifier* enables the user to correct the computer's data recognition errors before the data are sent to the database. In this step, the computer uses three methods to triangulate a level of confidence about the value of each response, and it indicates to the user if there is doubt about a particular item for data entry. In cases in which there is no doubt, the data fields in the database are approved automatically. Where there is doubt, the user is prompted to view a graphic image of the form in question and is shown the assumed value of the response. At this point, the user is able to edit the value so that the corrected value is the one entered into the database. Once all the corrections for the image have been made, the data are placed in the form's database.

There are no report writer functions in *Teleform*; therefore, the data must be exported to create reports. Several database formats can be chosen, including ASCII/text, dBase (1997), Microsoft Access (1996), FoxPro (1996), Paradox (1997), Microsoft Excel (1996), and SPSS (1996). From these formats, reports can be generated, or the data can be exported again and used with statistical analysis software programs such as SPSS or SAS.

Minimum system requirements include a Pentium base PC, 32 MB of RAM, and 100 MB of available hard drive space for software. In addition, a CD-ROM drive, one high-density 3.5-inch floppy disk drive, VGA color (or better) Windows-compatible monitor, mouse or other pointing device, Teleform-compatible scanner or fax-modem, laser or ink jet printer, and Windows 95 operating system are necessary (S. Baker, personal communication, January 12, 1998).

DEVELOPING AND MAINTAINING A SCANNABLE VARIANCE TRACKING SYSTEM

Variance tracking and analysis are essential components of health care management. We have defined a variance as any event that contributes to the acceleration or delay of an identified milestone, contributes to an avoidable day or phase in a patient's progress toward stated outcomes, or both. Variance tracking systems enable clinical teams to collect clinical data regarding whether or not a patient achieved an indicated outcome, identify factors that may explain variances of care, and provide information to guide care process redesign.

At St. Luke's, a work team was formed to develop a variance tracking system that was comprehensive, generic, customizable to meet various pathway-specific needs, low cost, reliable, and easy to use. The team consisted of staff with clinical expertise (therapist, clinical nurse specialist, staff nurse, and case manager) and expertise in data management and measurement (nurse researcher, quality management staff, and Clinical Information Services manager). The team's progress was periodically reported to the Quality Council, which was composed of representatives from administration, medical staff, and clinical staff.

We (the team members) agreed that the development of the variance tracking system needed to include domains of outcome variances; an outcome variance data dictionary; a valid, low-cost scannable variance tracking tool; a reliable process for tool use; data management procedures; and staff education on how to use the tool. The remainder of this chapter describes how we developed and currently maintain this variance tracking system.

CONCEPTUALIZING DOMAINS
OF OUTCOME VARIANCES

"Domains" of outcome variances are areas of behavior or experience that are characterized by specific features being measured. A review of the literature on outcome measurement and variance analysis revealed consistent inclusion of the following domains: delays related to patient and family, clinician and caregiver, hospital systems, and community resources. On the basis of some team members' previous experience with variance tracking, the domain of "variance acceleration" was also added. Our outcome variance tracking system has been in place for more than 1 year. The domains as originally conceptualized remain unchanged.

CREATING AND MAINTAINING A UNIFORM
OUTCOME VARIANCE DATA DICTIONARY

Our team brainstormed potential causes of variances within each of the domains based on a literature review and clinical expertise. When a variance cause was identified, we defined each variance category by consensus. Next, the variance categories and their definitions were sent to panels of experts from each discipline. These experts critiqued each term and definition until consensus was reached on the validity, clarity, and generalizability of each item of the uniform outcome variance data dictionary.

We recognized that two categories would need to have additional variances customized for each patient pathway: patient conditions that might cause a variance or abnormal diagnostic and lab tests unaddressed by caregivers that might cause a variance. Currently, each pathway team develops these variance labels and definitions with the same validation process as used by our original development team.

Once the outcome variance data dictionary was developed, the responsibility for maintenance of the dictionary was transferred to an accredited medical records specialist. This specialist maintains a master outcomes variance tracking data dictionary (Figure 6.1) that is used by pathway leaders when developing new pathways. Leaders are cautioned that there may be patient complications with the same variance label but with different code numbers and definitions within the master. For example, 215 (vomiting) is defined as "grade 3 or 4 per CALG-B toxicity criteria," whereas 227 (vomiting) is defined as "2-5 episodes of vomiting in 24 hours." Usually, the definitions for most variances can be found within the master dictionary, but leaders are given the latitude to add new labels and definitions to the master dictionary as needed.

DATA DICTIONARY FOR OUTCOMES VARIANCE CODES: Master

VARIANCE: Any event that contributes to the acceleration or delay of an identified milestone and/or contributes to an avoidable day or phase.
VARIANCE ACCELERATION: Patient achieves stated outcome or milestone sooner than the expected length of stay or phase in the following categories: **101 Patient/Family** **102 Clinician/Caregiver** **103 Hospital Systems** **104 Community Resources**
PATIENT/FAMILY

201 Indecision/Tests: Any patient and/or family who is undecided or refuses tests or treatments that result in an avoidable day/milestone.

202 Patient/Family Indecision/Discharge Planning: Any patient/family who is involved but fails in the decision making process related to discharge planning which results in an avoidable day/phase of stay.

203 Patient/Family Unavailable: Any patient/family that is not available and/or refuses to be available but is considered important to be present for teaching or discharge planning which results in an avoidable day/phase of stay.

204 Cultural, Health, Spiritual Beliefs: Any patient and/or family issues that delay the patient's progress due to cultural, health, or spiritual beliefs which results in an avoidable day/phase of stay.

205 Language Barrier: Any patient/family exhibit a language barrier that delays the patient's progress which results in an avoidable day/phase of stay.

206 Patient Participation in Education: Any patient that fails to participate in the education process or fails to carry out instruction in the process which results in a avoidable day/phase of stay.

207 Pathway Discontinued: Pathway no longer appropriate to guide plan of care (e.g. transfer to another level of care, death).

381 Cognitive Barrier: Limited ability of the mind to be aware of objects, thoughts or perceptions; includes all aspects of perceiving, thinking and remembering.

Conditions/Complications: Any unexpected physical and/or psychosocial patient condition/complication (e.g. unplanned surgical procedure, infection, coping deficit) defined by specific conditions/complications as listed below:

208 Other: Other physical and/or psychosocial patient complications not listed in variance codes below.

209 Nausea/Vomiting: Patient verbalizes nausea and/or vomiting and inability to tolerate diet.

210 Urinary Retention: Patient unable to void 6-8 hours post-operatively, requiring catheterization.

211 Fatigue/Decreased Endurance: Patient unable to participate in expected activities related to fatigue.

212 Pain: Patient indicates pain not controlled at acceptable level for patient.

213 Fatigue/Malaise: Defined as Grade 3 or 4 per CALG-B toxicity criteria.

214 Nausea: Defined as Grade 3 or 4 per CALG-B toxicity criteria.

215 Vomiting: Defined as Grade 3 or 4 per CALG-B toxicity criteria.

216 Neurotoxicity: Defined as Grade 3 or 4 per CALG-B toxicity criteria.

217 Diarrhea: Defined as Grade 3 or 4 per CALG-B toxicity criteria.

218 Mucositis/Stomatitis: Defined as Grade 3 or 4 per CALG-B toxicity criteria.

219 Dyspnea: Defined as Grade 3 or 4 per CALG-B toxicity criteria.

220 Atrial Fibrillation: Controlled or uncontrolled irregular cardiac arrhythmia characterized by chaotic atrial activity as seen on ECG or telemetry.

221 Pressure Ulcer: Any Stage II or greater lesion.

222 Fall with Injury: Any fall in which the patient suffers an abrasion, lesion, contusion, broken bone or decline in neurologic status.

223 Hemorrhage: Any significant ($\geq$50cc) external bleeding or internal bleeding as identified by lab or other diagnostic tests.

224 Cognitive Impairment: Patient unable to participate in expected activities related to cognitive impairment.

225 Fatigue/Malaise: Fatigue with impairment of ADLs.

226 Nausea: Intake significantly decreased, but can eat.

227 Vomiting: 2-5 episodes of vomiting in 24 hours.

228 Neurotoxicity: Moderate parasthesias, moderate somnolence or agitation.

229 Diarrhea: Increase of 4-6 stools/day, or nocturnal stools, or moderate cramping.

230 Mucositis/Stomatitis: Painful erythema, edema, or ulcers, but can eat.

231 Dyspnea: Respiratory difficulty at normal level of activity.

232 Nephrotoxicity: Creatinine level 1.5 - 3.0.

233 Hemodynamic Instability: Alterations in preload, afterload, heart rate, and/or contractility.

234 Preexisting Pulmonary Condition: Smoking (within 4 weeks prior to adm) &/or any of the following pulm conditions: COPD (chr obs asthma, chr obs bronchitis, ephysema, or chr airway obs), pulm embolism/infarct, acute cor pumonale/pulm HTN, pulm collapse, pulm fibrosis, or pleural effusion.

235 Sedation: Difficult to arrouse.

236 Neurological Compromise: Abnormal assessment findings: unable to follow commands, stroke, recent stroke, confusion, or neurological symptoms which limit the patient's ability to follow commands.

237 Respiratory Compromise: Abnormal lab or assessment findings including SAO2<90% on oxygen.

238 Other Cardiac Rhythm Disturbance: Symptomatic bradycardia, junctional rhythms, heart blocks (2nd or 3rd degree type), or

Figure 6.1. Master Data Dictionary for Outcomes Variance Codes (©1997, St. Luke's Medical Center, Milwaukee, Wisconsin. All Rights Reserved)

(Continued)

DATA DICTIONARY FOR OUTCOMES VARIANCE CODES: Master

ventricular dysrhythmias. (For atrial fibrillation, see code 220.)

239 **Atrial Fibrillation–Uncontrolled:** Postop onset of atrial fibrillation with uncontrolled ventricular rate > 100 bpm.

240 **Tongue Deviation:** Marked turning of tongue from the midline when protruded.

241 **Facial Paralysis:** Temporary or permanent loss of sensation or voluntary motion of the face.

242 **TIA:** Transient focal neurological deficit of vascular origin.

243 **Stroke:** Sudden severe episode of neurologial symptoms caused by a deficit in blood supply to the brain.

244 **Abnormal Blood Pressure:** Systolic blood pressure not in range 100-150.

245 **Hematoma:** Localized accumulation of blood, usually clotted in tissue due to break in a blood vessel wall that requires evacuation or surgical repair or impairs range of motion.

246 **Tamponade:** Acute compression of the heart due to effusion of fluid into the pericardium

247 **Lead Migration:** Movement of electrodes from their original pacing position

248 **Hemo/Pneumothorax:** Accumulation of air or blood in the pleural space, as a result of trauma.

249 **Rejection:** Myocardial biopsy results indicate pt is experiencing rejection, cellular (Grade II-III) and/or vascular

250 **Ileus:** Acute intestinal obstruction characterized by diminished or absent intestinal peristalsis, constipation, distention, abdominal pain and/or vomiting.

251 **Symptomatic Bradydysrhythmias:** Symptomatic bradycardia <50, junctional rhythms, heart blocks (2nd or 3rd degree type)

252 **Sinus Tachycardia:** >120 beats per minute.

253 **Ventricular Dysrhythmias:** Ventricular dysrhythmias requiring treatment with oral or IV medications, EP consult, etc.

254 **Ineffective Cough:** Failure to use abdominal muscles, cough generated from back of throat.

255 **Constipation:** No BM for 3 days, requires intervention to have stool.

CLINICIAN/CAREGIVER

301 **Delay the Initiation of Pathway:** Failure to initiate pathway within specified timeframe.

302 **Lack of Education:** Any situation in which there is insufficient education given to the patient and/or family which results in a avoidable day/phase of stay.

303 **Admission Criteria Not Met:** Intensity of service or severity of illness criteria not met on admission (UM).

304 **Continued Stay Criteria Not Met:** Extended LOS did not meet continued stay criteria (UM); e.g. outpatient procedure done as inpatient.

305 **Difficulty Contacting Physician:** Any situation where there was difficulty encountered in contacting a physician regarding orders that contributed to the delay of an identified or avoidable day/phase of stay.

306 **Procedure Delay/Medical Records:** Any situation in which care was delayed due to incomplete/unavailable medical records by a clinician/caregiver (e.g. H&P, Collaborative Database).

307 **Procedure Delay/Physician Request:** Any situation in which a procedure was delayed due to physician request.

308 **Procedure Delay/Communication:** Any situation in which a procedure was delayed due to a breakdown in communication that contributed to the delay of an identified milestone or avoidable day/phase of stay (e.g. physician-nurse, nurse-respiratory therapy.)

309 **Untimely Ancillary Referral:** Any situation resulting in an untimely referral that contributed to the delay of an identified milestone or an avoidable day/phase of stay.

310 **Untimely Physician to Physician Consultation:** Any situation resulting in an untimely consultation from physician to physician that contributed to the delay of an identified milestone or an avoidable day/phase of stay.

311 **Patient Not Seen within Established Timeframe:** Any situation in which a patient was not seen within established timeframe as per medical rules and regulations and/or unit or department policy that contributed to the delay of an identified milestone or avoidable day/phase of stay.

312 **D/C Orders Written Late:** Any situation that discharge orders are written late and D/C is delayed.

313 **Discharge/Transfer Delay: Medical Records Incomplete:** Any situation that the medical records were not completed or ready for discharge or transfer that caused a delay.

380 **Discharge/Transfer Delay: Physician Request:** Any situation in which a discharge or transfer was delayed due to physician request.

314 **Delay in Discharge Planning:** Any situation that caused a delay in discharge planning that contributed to the delay of identified milestone or avoidable day/phase of stay.

315 **Inadequate/Incorrect Prep:** Any situation that caused inadequate or incorrect preparation for procedure / test / intervention that contributed to the delay of an identified milestone or avoidable day/phase of stay.

316 **Incorrect Sequencing of Tests:** Any situation that caused incorrect sequencing of tests that contributed to the delay of an identified milestone or avoidable day/phase of stay (e.g. x-rays needed prior to treatment)

317 **Ordering Process Incorrect:** Any situation in which the ordering process was incorrect/incomplete that contributed to the delay of an identified milestone or avoidable day/phase of stay (e.g. wrong date/time, timeframe, incorrect test ordered)

Abnormal Physical Findings not Addressed: Any situation in which an abnormal diagnostic or lab test is not addressed that contributed to the delay of an identified milestone or avoidable day/phase:

318 **Other Abnormal Physical Findings Not Listed Below:** Other abnormal or lab tests not listed in Variance #s below:

319 **Low Hematocrit:** Hematocrit is less than 25

Figure 6.1. Continued

DATA DICTIONARY FOR OUTCOMES VARIANCE CODES: Master

320 Active Bleeding: Epistaxis; bleeding gums; blood in urine, stool, or emesis; severe petechiae or abnormal bruising.
321 Low Platelets: Platelets < 10,000 ul and refractory to platelet transfusions.
322 Low Hemoglobin: Hemoglobin < 8.0 gm/dl and refractory to transfusions.
323 Positive Cultures Indicating Infective Process: Positive cultures or oral temp > 101^F or chills.
324 Positive Radiology: Positive x-rays, CAT or nuclear medicine scans, MRI indicative of disease progression.
325 Positive Physical Findings: History of or assessment findings indicative of disease progression.
326 Interstitial Pneumonitis: Chest x-ray showing interstitial pneumonitis.
327 Low Hemoglobin: Hemoglobin < 8.5 gm/dl.
328 Low Platelets: Platelets < 10,000 µl.
329 Low WBC: WBC ≤ 2,000.
330 Low Platelets: Platelets < 50,000 µl.
331 Low Hemoglobin: Hemoglobin < 8 gm/dl.

HOSPITAL SYSTEMS

401 Scheduling Not Done on Weekends: Any occurrence in which test/treatment/intervention cannot be scheduled when requested due to scheduling not done on weekends that contributed to the delay of an identified milestone or avoidable day/phase of stay.
402 Scheduling Not Done on 2nd/3rd Shift: Any occurrence in which test/treatment/intervention cannot be scheduled when requested due to scheduling not done on 2nd/3rd shift that contributed to the delay of an identified milestone or avoidable day/phase of stay.
403 Department Closed: Any occurrence in which test/treatment/intervention cannot be scheduled when requested due to a department closure that contributed to the delay of an identified milestone or avoidable day/phase of stay.
404 No Openings in Schedule: Any occurrence in which test/procedure/intervention is delayed due lack of openings in the schedule that contributed to the delay of an identified milestone or avoidable day/phase of stay.
405 Equipment Failure/Unavailable: Any occurrence in which test/procedure intervention is delayed due to equipment failure or unavailability that contributed to the delay of an identified milestone or avoidable day/phase of stay.
406 Supplies Not Available: Any occurrence in which test/procedure/intervention was delayed due to unavailable supplies that contributed to the delay of an identified milestone or avoidable day/phase of stay.
407 Service Not Available at this Institution: Any occurrence in which test/procedure/intervention was delayed due to unavailable service at this institution that contributed to the delay of an identified milestone or avoidable day/phase of stay.
408 Computer Problems/Errors: Any occurrence where procedure/tests/admission/discharge or transfer is delayed due to computer problems/errors (e.g. computer down, upgrades) that contributed to the delay of an identified milestone or avoidable day/phase of stay.
409 Awaiting Hospital Bed/Unit: Any situation in which a patient transfer from a SLMC bed is delayed to another SLMC bed that contributed to the delay of an identified milestone or avoidable day/phase of stay (e.g., CVICU to 4/5LM.)
410 Medications Not Available: An ordered prescription/medication is not available at discharge pharmacy which causes any delay that contributed to the delay of an identified milestone or avoidable day/phase of stay.

COMMUNITY RESOURCES

501 Accepted, but No Bed/Service Available: Patient is accepted for admission to a non-SLMC service/bed but there is no bed/service available that contributed to the delay of an identified milestone or avoidable day/phase of stay (e.g. SNF, nursing home.)
502 Bed/Service Available, Facility would Not Accept Patient: Appropriate bed/service available but patient not accepted currently due to any reasons excluding financial/legal issues (e.g. patient/family behavior issues) that contributed to the delay of an identified milestone or avoidable day/phase of stay.
503 Durable Medical Equipment/Supplies Not Available: Durable medical equipment/supplies are not available due to reasons excluding insurance (e.g. demand exceeds supply, equipment not designed for home use) that contributed to the delay of an identified milestone or avoidable day/phase of stay.
504 Communication Breakdown Inside Aurora Affiliates: Any type of communication breakdown or miscommunication which results in a delay of admission/discharge/transfer among the Aurora affiliates (e.g. VNA, Bayshore Labs, AHM) that contributed to the delay of an identified milestone or avoidable day/phase of stay.
505 Communication Breakdown Outside Aurora: Any type of communication breakdown or miscommunication between SLMC and a non-Aurora agency/institution that results in a delay of admission/discharge/transfer that contributed to an identified milestone or avoidable day/phase of stay.
506 Financial/Legal Issues: Any situation which is due to a financial/legal or insurance related problem that results in a delay of discharge/transfer (e.g. awaiting guardianship; OBRA approval; insurance approval; 212 assignment) that contributed to the delay of an identified milestone or avoidable day/phase of stay.

Figure 6.1. Continued

DEVELOPING A VALID, LOW-COST, SCANNABLE VARIANCE TRACKING TOOL

Because our computerized patient record project was not due to be completed for 2 or 3 years, we needed to develop a temporary, low-cost option for variance tracking until we could abstract data from our automated system. Adding manual data entry responsibilities to our medical records (Clinical Information Services) staff was not possible because we were also undergoing organizational redesign to reduce overhead while maintaining quality. Therefore, we used Teleform Standard Version 5.3 and a Hewlett-Packard 4C Scanner to develop a low-cost, scannable variance tracking tool.

The component *Designer* was used to create a simple, customizable data collection tool to collect variance tracking data for all patient pathways. Our work team developed a generic template for the variance tracking form that consisted of nine sections: patient's medical record, patient's case number, patient pathway type, path day or phase, responsibility, outcome measure label, outcome number, codes for variance acceleration and delay, and directions for form completion. We experimented with various layouts until a simple, understandable format that accurately scanned 98% of the data was created. Figure 6.2 shows an example of the Outcome Variance Tracking Tool for the Inpatient CVA (cerebral vascular accident) pathway. An abbreviated version of the data dictionary for the Inpatient CVA is printed on the reverse side of the variance tracking tool (Figure 6.3), and a complete version of the data dictionary is laminated and available to staff as a reference on the units (Figure 6.4).

In this CVA example, the path day and outcome measures were modified on the template to indicate the first five patient outcome measures that the CVA patient pathway team decided to track. The selection of these specific outcome measures was based on the team members' clinical expertise of "critical" events that were essential to patients' progress toward outcome achievement. These outcome measures were reviewed by members of the multidisciplinary team's departments for validity and by the director of nursing research for clarity and congruence between the outcomes and the variance categories.

Figure 6.5 shows the CV surgery pathway variance tracking tool. In this pathway, the five outcome measures were selected based on a regression analysis of more than 40 daily outcome measures in more than 1,000 patients. These five criteria were independently the most predictive of patients' early discharge without complications. This pathway example shows how the template can be further modified to collect additional data the pathway teams deem to be important to understanding their process redesign. In this case type, we are now tracking data related to the time of patient arrival in the cardiovascular intensive care unit, extubation, and arrival to the intermediate care unit to better understand how we can further improve our patient outcomes. Teleform enables us to col-

Outcome Variance Tracking Tool
St. Luke's Medical Center
Milwaukee, Wisconsin

MRUN

MRU and Case Numbers are to be completed by Clinical Information Staff ONLY

Case#

0

HUC: *Stamp Here with Addressograph if Patient is on Inpatient CVA pathway*

Pathway

| 0 | 2 | **Inpatient CVA** |
Rev.1-6-98

Please form numbers as in the example below and avoid contact with the edge of the box.

0 1 2 3 4 5 6 7 8 9

Path Phase	Responsibility	Outcome Measure	Outcome Number	Variance
12-16 hrs post admit to unit	Speech Therapy	Swallow evaluation done	0 0 1	○ No Variance
Day 1	Nursing	NIH scoring done	0 0 2	○ No Variance
Day 2	Nursing	Physiatry evaluation done	0 0 3	○ No Variance
Day 2	PT/OT	Pt/family verbalize knowledge of: -Pt's sensory motor deficits -Plan for recovery	0 0 4	○ No Variance
Day 3	Social Services	Pt/family verbalize knowledge of pt's discharge disposition	0 0 5	○ No Variance

DIRECTIONS FOR FORM COMPLETION
1. *HUC stamps patient's addressograph in top right box of form.*
2. *Accountable departments review patient's achievement of daily/phase outcomes on the outcome due date, select the one MOST appropriate variance code (see laminated reference card), document variance code OR color in circle by "no variance" for each outcome by 2200.*
3. *The RN reviews the form daily and at discharge and notifies the Unit-Based OFT when incomplete data exist.*
4. *The Unit-Based OFT notifies the appropriate department to assure that data are recorded.*
5. *When the form is completed, it is left in the chart.*
   HUC sends completed form to Clinical Information Services with patient chart after discharge.
   Clinical Information Services staff verify MRU number, case number, and write in numbers in box on left top of form.
8. *Clinical Information Services staff scan and verify accurate data entry via Teleforms Verifier, then store form appropriately.*

Confidential QA/QI Document
DO NOT COPY!
To obtain additional copies, call your pathway team leader

22875

Figure 6.2. Inpatient CVA Outcome Variance Tracking Tool (©1997, St. Luke's Medical Center, Milwaukee, Wisconsin. All Rights Reserved)

lect text, numeric, multiple-choice, and date information to meet all our variance tracking needs.

We learned that it is important to duplicate each form from a master on a printshop-quality copy machine capable of producing 600 dots per inch resolu-

Variance Data Dictionary: Inpatient Cerebral Vascular Accident (CVA)

VARIANCE: Any event that contributes to the acceleration or delay of an identified milestone and/or contributes to an avoidable day or phase.

1. **Variance Acceleration**
   101 Patient / Family
   102 Clinician / Caregiver
   103 Hospital Systems
   104 Community Resources

2. **Patient / Family**
   201 Indecision / Tests
   202 Patient/Family Indecision / Discharge
   Planning
   203 Patient/Family Unavailable
   204 Cultural, Health, Spiritual Beliefs
   205 Language Barrier
   206 Patient Participation in Education
   207 Pathway Discontinued

   Complications
   208 Other
   220 Atrial Fibrillation
   221 Pressure Ulcer
   222 Fall with Injury
   223 Hemorrhage

3. **Clinician / Caregiver**
   301 Delay the Initiation of Pathway
   302 Lack of Education
   303 Admission Criteria not Met
   304 Continued Stay Criteria not Met
   305 Difficulty Contacting Physician
   306 Procedure Delay / Medical Records
   307 Procedure Delay / Physician Request
   308 Procedure Delay / Communication
   309 Untimely Ancillary Referral
   310 Untimely Physician to Physician
   Consultation
   311 Patient Not Seen w/in Established
   Timeframe
   312 D/C Orders Written Late
   313 Discharge/Transfer Delay: Medical
   Records Incomplete
   380 Discharge/Transfer Delay: Physician
   Request
   314 Delay in Discharge Planning
   315 Inadequate/Incorrect Prep
   316 Incorrect Sequencing of Tests
   317 Ordering Process Incorrect

Abnormal Physical Findings not Addressed
318 Other

4. **Hospital Systems**
   401 Scheduling Not Done on Weekends
   402 Scheduling Not Done on 2nd/3rd shift
   403 Department Closed
   404 No Openings in Schedule
   405 Equipment Failure/Unavailable
   406 Supplies Not Available
   407 Service Not Available at this Institution
   408 Computer Problems/Errors
   409 Awaiting Hospital Bed/Unit
   410 Medications Not Available

5. **Community Resources :**
   501 Accepted, but No Bed/Service Available
   502 Bed/service Available, Facility Would Not
   Accept Patient
   503 Durable Medical Equipment/Supplies Not
   Available
   504 Communication Breakdown/Aurora
   Affiliates
   505 Communication Breakdown/ Outside
   Aurora
   506 Financial/Legal Issues

Figure 6.3. Abbreviated Inpatient CVA Variance Data Dictionary (© 1997, St. Luke's Medical Center, Milwaukee, Wisconsin. All Rights Reserved)

DATA DICTIONARY FOR OUTCOMES VARIANCE CODES: Inpatient Cerebral Vascular Accident (CVA)

VARIANCE: Any event that contributes to the acceleration or delay of an identified milestone and/or contributes to an avoidable day or phase.

VARIANCE ACCELERATION: Patient achieves stated outcome or milestone sooner than the expected length of stay or phase in the following categories:

101 Patient/Family
102 Clinician/Caregiver
103 Hospital Systems
104 Community Resources

PATIENT/FAMILY

201 **Indecision/Tests:** Any patient and/or family who is undecided or refuses tests or treatments that result in an avoidable day/milestone.

202 **Patient/Family Indecision/Discharge Planning:** Any patient/family who is involved but fails in the decision making process related to discharge planning which results in an avoidable day/phase of stay.

203 **Patient/Family Unavailable:** Any patient/family that is not available and/or refuses to be available but is considered important to be present for teaching or discharge planning which results in an avoidable day/phase of stay.

204 **Cultural, Health, Spiritual Beliefs:** Any patient and/or family issues that delay the patient's progress due to cultural, health, or spiritual beliefs which results in an avoidable day/phase of stay.

205 **Language Barrier:** Any patient/family exhibit a language barrier that delays the patient's progress which results in an avoidable day/phase of stay.

206 **Patient Participation in Education:** Any patient that fails to participate in the education process or fails to carry out instruction in the process which results in a avoidable day/phase of stay.

207 **Pathway Discontinued:** Pathway no longer appropriate to guide plan of care (e.g. transfer to another level of care, death).

Conditions/Complications: Any unexpected physical and/or psychosocial patient condition/complication (e.g. unplanned surgical procedure, infection, coping deficit) defined by specific conditions/complications as listed below:

208 **Other:** Other physical and/or psychosocial patient complications not listed in variance codes below.

220 **Atrial Fibrillation:** Controlled or uncontrolled irregular cardiac arrhythmia characterized by chaotic atrial activity as seen on ECG or telemetry.

221 **Pressure Ulcer:** Any Stage II or greater lesion.

222 **Fall with Injury:** Any fall in which the patient suffers an abrasion, lesion, contusion, broken bone or decline in neurologic status.

223 **Hemorrhage:** Any significant ($\geq$50cc) external bleeding or internal bleeding as identified by lab or other diagnostic tests.

CLINICIAN/CAREGIVER

301 **Delay the Initiation of Pathway:** Failure to initiate pathway within specified timeframe.

302 **Lack of Education:** Any situation in which there is insufficient education given to the patient and/or family which results in a avoidable day/phase of stay.

303 **Admission Criteria Not Met:** Intensity of service or severity of illness criteria not met on admission (UM).

304 **Continued Stay Criteria Not Met:** Extended LOS did not meet continued stay criteria (UM); e.g. outpatient procedure done as inpatient.

305 **Difficulty Contacting Physician:** Any situation where there was difficulty encountered in contacting a physician regarding orders that contributed to the delay of an identified or avoidable day/phase of stay.

306 **Procedure Delay/Medical Records:** Any situation in which care was delayed due to incomplete/unavailable medical records by a clinician/caregiver (e.g. H&P, Collaborative Database).

307 **Procedure Delay/Physician Request:** Any situation in which a procedure was delayed due to physician request.

308 **Procedure Delay/Communication:** Any situation in which a procedure was delayed due to a breakdown in communication that contributed to the delay of an identified milestone or avoidable day/phase of stay (e.g. physician-nurse, nurse-respiratory therapy.)

309 **Untimely Ancillary Referral:** Any situation resulting in an untimely referral that contributed to the delay of an identified milestone or an avoidable day/phase of stay.

310 **Untimely Physician to Physician Consultation:** Any situation resulting in an untimely consultation from physician to physician that contributed to the delay of an identified milestone or an avoidable day/phase of stay.

311 **Patient Not Seen within Established Timeframe:** Any situation in which a patient was not seen within established timeframe as per medical rules and regulations and/or unit or department policy that contributed to the delay of an identified milestone or avoidable day/phase of stay.

312 **D/C Orders Written Late:** Any situation that discharge orders are written late and D/C is delayed.

313 **Discharge/Transfer Delay: Medical Records Incomplete:** Any situation that the medical records were not completed or ready for discharge or transfer that caused a delay.

380 **Discharge/Transfer Delay: Physician Request:** Any situation in which a discharge or transfer was delayed due to physician request.

314 **Delay in Discharge Planning:** Any situation that caused a delay in discharge planning that contributed to the delay of identified milestone or avoidable day/phase of stay.

315 **Inadequate/Incorrect Prep:** Any situation that caused inadequate or incorrect preparation for procedure / test / intervention that contributed to the delay of an identified milestone or avoidable day/phase of stay.

Figure 6.4. Data Dictionary for Outcomes Variance Codes: Inpatient CVA
(© 1997, St. Luke's Medical Center, Milwaukee, Wisconsin. All Rights Reserved)

(Continued)

DATA DICTIONARY FOR OUTCOMES VARIANCE CODES: Inpatient Cerebral Vascular Accident (CVA)

316 **Incorrect Sequencing of Tests:** Any situation that caused incorrect sequencing of tests that contributed to the delay of an identified milestone or avoidable day/phase of stay (e.g. x-rays needed prior to treatment)

317 **Ordering Process Incorrect:** Any situation in which the ordering process was incorrect/incomplete that contributed to the delay of an identified milestone or avoidable day/phase of stay (e.g. wrong date/time, timeframe, incorrect test ordered)

Abnormal Physical Findings not Addressed: Any situation in which an abnormal diagnostic or lab test is not addressed that contributed to the delay of an identified milestone or avoidable day/phase:

318 **Other Abnormal Physical Findings Not Listed Below:** Other abnormal or lab tests not listed in Variance #s below:

HOSPITAL SYSTEMS

401 **Scheduling Not Done on Weekends:** Any occurrence in which test/treatment/intervention cannot be scheduled when requested due to scheduling not done on weekends that contributed to the delay of an identified milestone or avoidable day/phase of stay.

402 **Scheduling Not Done on 2nd/3rd Shift:** Any occurrence in which test/treatment/intervention cannot be scheduled when requested due to scheduling not done on 2nd/3rd shift that contributed to the delay of an identified milestone or avoidable day/phase of stay.

403 **Department Closed:** Any occurrence in which test/treatment/intervention cannot be scheduled when requested due to a department closure that contributed to the delay of an identified milestone or avoidable day/phase of stay.

404 **No Openings in Schedule:** Any occurrence in which test/procedure/intervention is delayed due to equipment failure or unavailability that contributed to the delay of an identified milestone or avoidable day/phase of stay.

405 **Equipment Failure/Unavailable:** Any occurrence in which test/procedure intervention is delayed due to equipment failure or unavailability that contributed to the delay of an identified milestone or avoidable day/phase of stay.

406 **Supplies Not Available:** Any occurrence in which test/procedure/intervention was delayed due to unavailable supplies that contributed to the delay of an identified milestone or avoidable day/phase of stay.

407 **Service Not Available at this Institution:** Any occurrence in which test/procedure/intervention was delayed due to unavailable service at this institution that contributed to the delay of an identified milestone or avoidable day/phase of stay.

408 **Computer Problems/Errors:** Any occurrence where procedure/tests/admission/discharge or transfer is delayed due to computer problems/errors (e.g. computer down, upgrades) that contributed to the delay of an identified milestone or avoidable day/phase of stay.

409 **Awaiting Hospital Bed/Unit:** Any situation in which a patient transfer from a SLMC bed is delayed to another SLMC bed that contributed to the delay of an identified milestone or avoidable day/phase of stay (e.g., CVICU to 4/5LM.)

410 **Medications Not Available:** An ordered prescription/medication is not available at discharge pharmacy which causes any delay that contributed to the delay of an identified milestone or avoidable day/phase of stay.

COMMUNITY RESOURCES

501 **Accepted, but No Bed/Service Available:** Patient is accepted for admission to a non-SLMC service/bed but there is no bed/service available that contributed to the delay of an identified milestone or avoidable day/phase of stay (e.g. SNF, nursing home.)

502 **Bed/Service Available, Facility would Not Accept Patient:** Appropriate bed/service available but patient not accepted currently due to any reasons excluding financial/legal issues (e.g. patient/family behavior issues) that contributed to the delay of an identified milestone or avoidable day/phase of stay.

503 **Durable Medical Equipment/Supplies Not Available:** Durable medical equipment/supplies are not available due to reasons excluding insurance (e.g. demand exceeds supply, equipment not designed for home use) that contributed to the delay of an identified milestone or avoidable day/phase of stay.

504 **Communication Breakdown Inside Aurora Affiliates:** Any type of communication breakdown or miscommunication which results in a delay of admission/discharge/transfer among the Aurora affiliates (e.g. VNA, Bayshore Labs, AHM) that contributed to the delay of an identified milestone or avoidable day/phase of stay.

505 **Communication Breakdown Outside Aurora:** Any type of communication breakdown or miscommunication between SLMC and a non-Aurora agency/institution that results in a delay of admission/discharge/transfer that contributed to the delay of an identified milestone or avoidable day/phase of stay.

506 **Financial/Legal Issues:** Any situation which is due to a financial/legal or insurance related problem that results in a delay of discharge/transfer (e.g. awaiting guardianship; OBRA approval; insurance approval; 212 assignment) that contributed to the delay of an identified milestone or avoidable day/phase of stay.

Figure 6.4. Continued

Figure 6.5. CV Surgery Outcome Variance Tracking Tool (©1997, St. Luke's Medical Center, Milwaukee, Wisconsin. All Rights Reserved)

tion. This high-quality resolution enables the scanner to accurately identify and place data during the scanning process. We also learned to emphasize to the staff not to copy these forms on unit-based copy machines because some copiers create blurred copies. When these blurred copies are scanned, the data are not recognizable by the scanner, and additional manual data entry is necessary.

The variance tracking forms are printed on yellow paper to facilitate Clinical Information Services staff's easy recognition and retrieval of the forms from the medical record when the record is sent down for final storage. We have had no problems with scanning forms on colored paper, but we have avoided bright colors to enhance data recognition.

CREATING AND MAINTAINING A RELIABLE PROCESS FOR TOOL USE

The clinical staff members of the work team negotiated the responsibilities of who should fill out the forms, when the forms should be completed, and who should send the forms to Clinical Information Services. Once these issues were resolved, the directions for form completion were added to the variance tracking form template (see the bottom of Figures 6.2 or 6.5).

To ensure that the form was consistently and accurately being completed according to the guidelines, the pathway leaders (usually clinical nurse specialists or expert staff nurses) select 10 charts by convenience sampling during the initial month of implementation. They review the patient's progress daily and rate the patient's achievement of the outcome measures independently from the patient's caregivers. During our first year, we found that interrater reliability estimates between the team leaders and the staff for each item ranged from 0% to 100%. When interrater reliability is low (<80%), pathway teams clarify outcome measures or provide additional caregiver training or both. We recommend that team leaders routinely conduct this interrater reliability check when introducing a new pathway or a new outcome criteria.

IDENTIFYING AND MAINTAINING DATA MANAGEMENT PROCEDURES

Variance tracking tools are placed on the patient's chart by the staff on the admitting nursing unit. Staff accountable for documenting outcome achievement either write in the variance acceleration or delay code or color in the bubble next to "no variance" for each outcome measure on the indicated path day. The forms are kept in a binder for use by outcomes facilitation teams during daily rounds. These teams (composed of the staff nurse, manager, clinical nurse specialist, and social worker [routinely] and therapists, nutritionists, pharmacists, and physicians when available) complete the forms as appropriate daily. A unit secretary places them in the patient's chart and sends the chart to Clinical Information Services at discharge. Clinical Information Services staff remove the forms from the charts when the patient is discharged.

The Clinical Information Services staff verify the patient's medical record and case numbers on the patient addressograph against hospital information system databases and record the numbers on the variance tracking form. Weekly, the forms are scanned into the computer and verified by one of the Clinical Information Services staff (a high school graduate who is comfortable working with computers—not a registered medical records specialist). On a monthly basis, a clinical data specialist imports the Teleform variance tracking data into a FoxPro database, in which they are linked with demographic (age and gender), clinical (comorbidities and length of stay), and financial (charge) data from ChartStat (1997) and cost data from Transitional Systems, Inc. (1997; another financial database). Next, summary reports are generated using R&R Report Writer (1995).

The variance analysis reports are sent to the team leaders, who share them with the team members for review and action. Figure 6.6 shows a sample of the report sent to the Inpatient CVA team leader in December 1997. These data have been helpful in identifying the need to have more consistent staff documentation of variances and the need to explore reasons for delays in completing physiatry evaluations according to the pathway time frame.

CREATING AN EDUCATIONAL PROCESS FOR STAFF ON HOW TO USE THE TOOL

Whenever a new pathway is introduced into an area that has not previously been educated on patient pathways, a portion of the educational program is used to show staff how to initiate and complete the variance tracking tool. The form is shown, and the directions for form completion at the bottom are reviewed. The staff are provided with a case scenario and shown how a completed variance tracking form looks. Once the patient pathway and variance tracking forms are introduced on the clinical units, outcome facilitation teams review the patient's progress each day and ensure that the variance tracking forms are completed accurately. If staff knowledge deficits are identified, individual educational sessions are provided.

EVALUATING THE VARIANCE TRACKING PROCESS

In postimplementation focus groups, physicians reported satisfaction with consistently receiving data on how care processes can be improved on a monthly basis. Staff reported that the variance tracking tool is simple, clear, and easy to use. Staff appreciated having to document only five key outcome measures identified by the pathway teams rather than tracking each process step and patient outcome.

November, 1997 Outcomes Variance Report for Inpatient CVA Pathway
16 cases

Outcome Measure # 1: Swallowing evaluation done

Variance Code	Category & Description	Count	%
307	Clinician/Caregiver: Procedure delay/ Physician Request	2	12.50
308	Clinician/Caregiver: Procedure delay/ Communication	1	6.25
311	Clinician/Caregiver: Patient not seen within established timeframe	1	6.25
Blank	No entry made for this outcome	7	43.75
No variance	No variance	5	31.25

Outcome Measure # 2: NIH scoring done

Variance Code	Category & Description	Count	%
201	Patient/Family: Indecision/Tests	1	6.25
311	Clinician/Caregiver: Patient not seen within established time frame	1	6.25
Blank	No entry made for this outcome	2	12.50
No variance	No variance	12	75.00

Outcome Measure # 3: Physiatry evaluation done

Variance Code	Category & Description	Count	%
202	Patient/Family: Patient/family indecision/ Discharge planning	1	6.25
307	Clinician/Caregiver: Physician request	6	37.50
Blank	No entry made for this outcome	6	37.50
No variance	No variance	3	18.75

Outcome Measure # 4: Patient/family verbalize knowledge of patient's sensory motor deficits, plan for recovery AND Outcome Measure # 5: Patient/family verbalize knowledge of patient's discharge disposition

Variance Code	Category & Description	Count	%
Blank	No entry made for this outcome	13	81.25
No variance	No variance	3	18.75

Figure 6.6. November 1997 Outcomes Variance Report for Inpatient CVA Pathway (© 1997, St. Luke's Medical Center, Milwaukee, Wisconsin. All Rights Reserved)

Our most significant problem is missing data. In focus groups, staff indicated that there were a variety of reasons for the missing data, but the most common ones were "lack of time" and "low on my priority list." Several staff have commented that this problem will decrease when variance data are abstracted electronically from data that are routinely entered in the patients' computerized records.

Pathway team leaders were asked to comment on the variance tracking process and outcomes for this chapter. Cindy Lewis, RN, MSN, clinical nurse specialist, and team leader of the carotid endarterectomy pathway responded as follows:

> The data I receive from variance tracking have been extremely helpful in evaluating our present care and practice. These data will drive further practice changes and identify future practice needs. It would be nice if the monthly information could be charted on control charts with control limits to show how we are doing over time with each outcome measure. Quality management is helping to format the data this way for staff.

The Clinical Information Services staff also reported being able to manage large volumes of variance tracking data at significantly lower cost because of their ability to bypass manual data entry.

SUMMARY

In all our pathways, the outcome facilitation teams have used the variance tracking data to identify areas for further process improvement. Thus, this variance analysis system, using low-cost scanning technology, has met the initial objectives of being comprehensive, generic, customizable to meet various pathway-specific needs, low cost, reliable, and easy to use.

REFERENCES

Access [Computer software]. (1996). Redmond, WA: Microsoft.

ChartStat [Computer software]. (1997). Bethesda, MD: SoftMed Systems.

dBase [Computer software]. (1997). Scotts Valley, CA: Borland.

Excel [Computer software]. (1996). Redmond, WA: Microsoft.

FoxPro [Computer software]. (1996). Redmond, WA: Microsoft.

Paradox [Computer software]. (1997). Scotts Valley, CA: Borland.

R&R report writer [Computer software]. (1995). Westborough, MA: Concentric Data Systems.

Smyth, E. T., McIlvenny, G., Barr, J. G., Dickson, L. M., & Thompson, I. M. (1997). Automated entry of hospital infection surveillance data. *Infection Control & Hospital Epidemiology, 18*(7), 486-491.

SPSS 7.5 for Windows [Computer software]. (1996). Chicago: SPSS.

Teleform standard Version 5.3 [Computer software]. (1997). San Marcos, CA: Cardiff Software.

Transitional systems, Inc. [Computer software]. (1997). Boston: Transitional Systems.

FURTHER READING

Davidson, L. J., Ryan, W. J., Rohay, J. M., & Sereika, S. M. (1996). Technological advances in data entry and verification: Is Teleform for you? *Nursing Research, 45*(6), 373-376.

Dennis, K. E. (1994). Managing questionnaire data through optical scanning technology. *Nursing Research, 43,* 376-378.

Gerber, R. M., Atwood, J. R., Hinshaw, A. S., & Erickson, J. R. (1986). Optical scanning and computer technology in nursing research. *Computers in Nursing, 4,* 241-245.

Hammer, J. S., Strain, J. J., & Lyerly, M. (1993). An optical scan/statistical package for clinical data management in C-L psychiatry. *General Hospital Psychiatry, 15*(2), 95-101.

Jensen, P. S., Irwin, R. A., Josephson, A. M., Davis, H., Xenakis, S. N., Bloedau, L., Ness, R., Mabem A., Lee, B., Traylor, J., & Clawson, L. (1996). Data-gathering tools for "real world" clinical settings: A multisite feasibility study. *Journal of the American Academy of Child & Adolescent Psychiatry, 35,* 55-66.

Nolan, M. T., Nyberg, D. M., Poe, S. S., Case-Cromer, D., Frink, B. B., Schauble, J. F., & Paul, S. (1997). Scanner technology for data-based decision making. *Nursing Economics, 15,* 24-31.

PART II

Case Studies in Patient Outcomes Management

EDITORS' NOTE: Those responsible for managing patient outcomes need to identify factors that contribute to negative outcomes and work within the multidisciplinary group to improve care. How is this accomplished in the acute care setting when the negative outcome does not occur until after discharge and the contributing factors occur in three different locations during the hospitalization? This chapter describes how Research Nurse Program Coordinator Maura Goldsborough worked with case managers and the multidisciplinary team in the operating room, critical care unit, general care unit, and home care services to study factors that contribute to leg graft wound infections following coronary artery bypass graft. If you think that a project that involves many people, multiple locations, volumes of data, and practice changes sounds daunting, read on.

Factors Associated With Leg Graft Wound Complications Following Coronary Artery Bypass

Maura A. Goldsborough

IDENTIFYING THE PATIENT OUTCOME

Coronary artery bypass grafting is currently the most frequently performed surgical procedure in the United States, with more than 400,000 patients undergoing surgery during 1996. Although the surgical mortality has remained low, 2% or 3% (Katz & Chase, 1997), the associated morbidity with this procedure, including stroke and infection, has ranged from 5% to 19% (Shuhaiber, Chugh, Portoian-Shuhaiber, & Ghosh, 1987; Townsend, Reitz, Bilker, & Bartlett, 1993; Wells, Newsom, & Rowlands, 1983). At The Johns Hopkins Hospital in Baltimore, the incidence and factors associated with coronary artery bypass outcomes such as stroke have been well described (McKhann, Goldsborough, & Borowicz, 1997). Morbidity associated with leg graft wound infections, however, has not been clearly studied. This may be due in part to the changing health care environment. Because patients are being discharged sooner following surgery, more postoperative complications are occurring at home. This change in environment presents a new challenge to nurse clinicians seeking to manage and prevent these complications. Identification of the incidence and factors associated with selected patient outcomes can help to provide continuity of care and ensure that changes in health care delivery do not adversely affect morbidity.

Since 1980, only a few studies have examined the incidence of leg wound complications. Previous reports found incidences of leg graft wound infections from 2% to 19% (Gentry, Zeluff, & Cooley, 1988; Wells et al., 1983). The three studies with the largest number of patients were completed to determine the efficacy of different antibiotics (Conklin et al., 1988; Gentry et al., 1988; Townsend et al., 1993). Of the studies completed, few have identified factors associated with these leg wound problems.

Therefore, the purpose of our project was to identify the incidence of leg graft wound complications in patients undergoing coronary artery bypass grafting at our institution. We were also interested in determining whether we could identify factors associated with the standard intraoperative or postoperative care that contributed to leg graft complications.

BUILDING THE TEAM

This project was initiated by the nurse case managers who manage the care of patients having cardiac surgery both in the immediate postoperative hospitalization and during the first few weeks following discharge. They elicited help from me, the research nurse program coordinator for cardiac surgery, to serve as the project leader. During the spring of 1994, it was noted that many patients were calling the case managers from home and stating that they were having leg wound complications. This meant that the patient would have to travel back to the hospital for the case managers to assess the leg wound and determine the necessary intervention. Although during the first 2 weeks of surgery patients are mobile enough to travel, they are not able to drive. Therefore, a family member or caregiver needed to drive the patient back to the hospital clinic setting. A significant amount of the case managers' time was then devoted to meeting with patients and their families in the clinic.

The goal of case management is to maximize the quality and efficiency of the care delivered. In 1994, at our institution improvement in care processes led to shorter hospital stays. Whereas in the past patients were still hospitalized when leg wound problems occurred, patients were now in the home setting. We immediately realized that to accomplish our goal of identifying the incidence and factors associated with leg wound complications we needed to extend our data collection into the postdischarge period. This required collaboration with home health care nurses and increased levels of communication with patients and families following hospital discharge.

Therefore, it was clear that a multidiciplinary approach to this project was required. The project team included a research nurse program coordinator, operating room nurses, intensive care unit nurses, cardiac surgery case managers, and various home health care nurses from multiple home health agencies. By incorporating such a vast range of nursing personnel, we were able to maximize the information collected. We also thought it was important to include all personnel on our surgery team, including surgeons and physician assistants, because we would be examining their practice in the operating room. We met with the surgical teams at the beginning of our project to explain what leg problems were occurring and the goals of our project. We received their support from the outset. The data that were to be collected were discussed with the surgical team, and their input was included in the planning and data collection. By using this collaborative approach, we avoided possible conflicts as the project progressed.

During the initial phase of our project, we needed to assess the existing information we had concerning leg wound problems. Unfortunately, we realized that this information was not collected in a standardized way but rather recorded anecdotally. Therefore, we needed to determine a mechanism for identifying leg wound problems for both inpatients and outpatients within our institution. Next, we needed to formulate a plan for how we would collect the information on patients' hospital courses and who would need to be involved to complete the project. By determining the data we wanted to collect in the initial phases, we were able to identify which nursing personnel would need to play roles in the project. The roles of the team participants are summarized in the following sections.

Research Nurse Program Coordinator

The research nurse played a primary role in the project. This nurse was able to assist in data collection, data entry, and data analysis. The responsibilities included designing the data collection tool. Because we knew that many persons would be involved in the data collection, the tool needed to be simple to read and easy to use. In addition, it was necessary for the research nurse to elicit feedback from the surgeons and physician assistants to determine if any other information was necessary to make this project complete. Next, the research nurse was responsible for getting the data collection tools from the operating room setting to the intensive care unit. An essential part of the project was coordinating additional data collection with the case managers for patients who eventually had a leg wound complication. The final responsibility of the research nurse was to review the findings of this project with all the staff involved and to serve as lead author in the publication of these findings (Goldsborough et al., 1999).

Operating Room Nurses

These nurses were responsible for starting the data collection tool and for documenting critical information on operative care for each patient. They also started the documentation on patients' medical histories. The study team asked the operating room nurses to collect information that was not a routine part of their clinical documentation. This information proved to be critical to our project. The nurse manager of the operating room played an integral part by assisting in the orientation of the nurses. She provided inservices to the staff on how to complete the data tool and assisted in coordination of these nurses during the entire project.

Intensive Care Unit Nurses

The nurses in our intensive care unit (ICU) take great pride in the care they give their patients. For years, they have maintained a high standard of care. They were aware that there was a possibility that their routine of care would be scrutinized by this project. Before we started data collection, our study team met with the ICU nurses to explain the purpose of the project. They willingly agreed to join our project and assist in data collection on a daily basis. Our initial plan was to examine the routine medications and incision site care that was administered within the first 24 to 48 hours postoperatively to our coronary artery bypass patients.

Case Managers

Once the patients leave the ICU, they come under the care of the case managers, who typically follow patients while hospitalized until they are discharged home. In the past, most patients were discharged on Postoperative Day 7. With the onset of managed care, however, the target day for discharge has become Day 5 or 6. Therefore, the case managers' role now extends into the community when patients return home.

Patients and families were educated on the signs and symptoms of infection before discharge (both by the nurse at the bedside and by videotape) and were instructed to report any signs and symptoms of infections to either the nursing staff or the medical staff at our institution. This became a critical mechanism for identifying leg wound infections that occurred in the community or home setting.

Home Health Care Nurses

The majority of patients who leave the hospital in 5 or 6 days have a visit from a home health care nurse, at which time the integrity of the incision sites is assessed. If patients had signs and symptoms of complications with the leg incisions, the home health care nurses would contact the case managers at our institution, who then saw the patient in the clinic to fully assess the problems.

SELECTING THE INSTRUMENTS

The decision about what data to collect was made on a multidisciplinary level. In addition to considering factors that typically lead to infection, such as diabetes mellitus and use of steroids, we challenged ourselves to think of routine clinical practice issues that might have an impact on patient outcomes.

The data tool was structured in three sections: preoperative and demographic factors, intraoperative factors, and postoperative factors. In designing the data tool, we realized immediately that surgical personnel who performed the leg incision might feel uncomfortable with our data acquisition. We therefore decided at the outset to include the physician assistants and surgeons in our plans for this project. We reviewed the data points we were going to collect, and we included all the surgical personnel in this review. We asked them if they had any ideas about additional data we should collect. This turned out to be the most important interaction we had in our planning phase, and we effectively avoided a potential barrier to the completion of our project. The additional variables that were suggested to us by the physician assistants turned out to be the most critical data that were gathered.

The final data collection tool included all the variables shown in Tables 7.1, 7.2, and 7.3. One problem with this tool was that because the operating room nurses were the starting point or initiators of the tool, data that were missed in the operating room were essentially lost to us. Weekly data reports were checked by the research nurse for completeness. Reports to the nurse manager of the operating room were made to correct these missing data points throughout the project. Thus, the data tool and data collection were truly a group effort.

MEASURING THE PATIENT OUTCOME

It was decided from the outset of our project that we wanted to collect information on any patients who had any complaint of leg complications postoperatively, regardless of the need for intervention. All complications required the attention of the case managers and physicians on the cardiac team. Therefore, we defined our outcome as any postoperative leg wound complication.

Leg complications were identified during both hospitalization and post-hospital discharge. It was interesting that some patients who appeared to be fine while hospitalized developed complications while at home. This was one of the first surgical projects at our institution that encompassed outcomes that

TABLE 7.1 Relationships Between Preoperative Factors and Leg Wound Complications[a]

Factor	No Leg Problems: n (%)	Leg Problems: n (%)
Number of patients	510 (93)	37 (7)
Mean age	65.2	64.3
Gender		
Male	348 (68)	23 (62)
Female	162 (32)	14 (38)
Hospitalized preoperatively	206 (40)	9 (24)*
Recent smoking history	302 (59)	18 (49)
Diabetes mellitus	146 (29)	12 (32)
Peripheral vascular disease	92 (18)	8 (22)
Past vascular surgery	59 (12)	5 (14)
Steroid use	18 (4)	3 (8)
Past deep vein thrombosis	16 (3)	1 (3)
Leg edema	49 (12)	6 (21)
Mean body surface area (M^2)	1.93	1.94

a. t Test was used for continuous variables, and chi-square analysis was used for categorical variables.
*$p < .01$.

TABLE 7.2 Relationships Between Intraoperative Factors and Leg Wound Complications[a]

Factor	No Leg Problems: n (%)	Leg Problems: n (%)
Number of patients	510 (93)	37 (7)
Ace bandage wrapping	80 (17)	10 (33)*
Cardiopulmonary bypass (minutes)	119	128*
Time leg was open (minutes)	110	144*
Continuous incision	124 (25)	14 (38)*
Intraaortic ballon pump	48 (10)	5 (14)
Drain used	19 (4)	3 (9)
Leg irrigated	483 (98)	33 (94)
Femoral sheath	40 (8)	4 (11)
Cautery	31 (7)	2 (7)
Dura-prep	134 (27)	12 (32)
Betadine prep	22 (4)	2 (5)
Betadine/alcohol prep	350 (69)	23 (62)
Number of coronary grafts	3.2	3.4
Aortic cross-clamp time (minutes)	74	76

a. t Test was used for continuous variables, and chi-square analysis was used for categorical variables.
*$p < .01$.

TABLE 7.3 Relationships Between Postoperative Factors and Leg Wound Complications[a]

Factor	No Leg Problems: n (%)	Leg Problems: n (%)
Number of patients	510 (93)	37 (7)
Intravenous drug administered		
Epinephrine	58 (12)	9 (24)*
Nitroglycerine	367 (73)	18 (49)*
Nicardipine	25 (5)	5 (14)*
Dobutamine	85 (17)	2 (5)*
Dopamine	396 (79)	30 (81)
Nitroprusside	330 (66)	20 (54)
Neosynephrine	20 (4)	1 (3)
Levophed	5 (1)	0 (0)
Inocor	20 (4)	3 (8.1)
Fluid gained (kilograms)	5.0	5.8

a. t Test was used for continuous variables, and chi-square analysis was used for categorical variables.
*$p < .01$.

occurred both in the hospital and following discharge. The research nurse was responsible for entering and managing the data. This was done using a personal computer with a relational database program (Paradox, 1998).

ANALYZING THE DATA

The initial step in our data analysis focused on our outcome, which was a leg wound complication. We asked the following yes-or-no question: Did the patient have a leg wound complication? Thus, our outcome was dichotomous. As a first attempt, we examined the data on a univariate level—that is, we examined each variable by itself in relation to the outcome. For example, we asked the following question: Is this variable (diabetes) statistically significant in relation to developing a leg wound complication? Two statistical tests were used in this phase of data analysis: Student's t test and chi-square (Visintainer, 1986).

For variable questions that could be answered yes or no, such as the diabetes question, the chi-square test was used. For variables that are continuous, such as age, the Student's t test was used. Tables 7.1, 7.2, and 7.3 summarize the relationships between leg wound complications and factors in the preoperative, intraoperative, and postoperative periods. Using these tests allowed statistical significance to be determined for each individual variable.

We then conducted additional analyses. Factors that were found to be significant in the univariate analysis (t test and chi-square) were combined. By combining these factors using multiple logistic regression, the most important group of factors emerged and we were able to calculate the odds ratios. This type of analysis allows the factors that are most important to be determined when examining all the factors together. We carried out a variety of steps for the logistic regression analysis to help us to better understand the factors that we could use to change our practice.

SUMMARIZING THE FINDINGS

Using logistic regression, we were able to reduce the number of factors that were important to the outcome of leg wound complication (Table 7.4). In the final step of the analysis, we discovered that only one of the preoperative factors was important. However, events that occurred in the operating room and in the ICU were critical to patient outcome. The use of a calcium channel blocker in the ICU and the amount of time the leg incision was open during the operation were significantly related to the development of a problem. It was immediately clear that we could impact these problems by making changes in routine clinical care.

APPLYING THE FINDINGS TO PRACTICE

The results of this project had a large impact on our routine clinical practice. The most interesting result of our project was that factors that we initially thought would predispose patients to leg wound complications were not the factors we found to be important. For example, patients who were diabetic or were taking steroids before surgery were not found to be at higher risk. The results indicated that the events that occurred once patients were in the health care system were significant.

The only preoperative factor found to be significant was whether or not patients were hospitalized immediately before their surgery. We hypothesized that this might be related to the increased infection potential of hospitalized patients and potential inadequacies with preoperative scrubbing and cleansing in the hospitalized population. This was believed to be a serious issue for nursing care and nursing education in the preoperative period. Subsequent staff inservices have been completed to ensure the adequacy of these practices.

In terms of intraoperative factors, one of the most significant factors for leg wound complications was the amount of time that the leg incision was open during the surgical procedure. This variable was suggested as important at the start of the project by the physician assistants. This finding would directly affect their practice. We sought to change this behavior of prolonging the time the leg incision was open in the operating room. It was reported that at times the surgeon would ask the physician assistant for help in the chest surgical field. If the leg wound were not yet closed, the physician assistant would cover it with a sterile

TABLE 7.4 Relationships Between Factors at All Periods and Leg Wound Complications

Factor	Time Period	Odds Ratio
Step 1. All significant variables included		
Not on dobutamine	Post-op	7.4*
On nircardipine	Post-op	4.3*
Hospitalized preoperatively	Pre-op	3.5**
Use of ace bandage wrapping	Intra-op	3.2**
Not on nitroglycerin	Post-op	3.0**
Time leg was open	Intra-op	1.0**
Step 2. Time leg was open used as a dichotomous variable		
Not on dobutamine	Post-op	8.4*
On nicardipine	Post-op	3.7*
Not on nitroglycerin	Post-op	3.4**
Leg open >150 minutes	Intra-op	2.6**

$*p < .05; **p < .01.$

towel until able to return to close the site. Currently, the leg incision is closed as quickly as possible in an effort to minimize leg incision complications.

Another intraoperative factor found to be important was the use of an ace bandage wrapping on the leg incision at the conclusion of the surgery. The leg incision was wrapped to assist in reducing the swelling at the site. This was usually done for a subset of patients by surgeon preference. Use of this leg wrapping increased the patients' risk of developing a leg wound complication. As a result of our finding, this technique is no longer used at our institution.

The postoperative factor found to be significant was the use of intravenous medications. We did not fully understand at first how medications might contribute to a leg wound complication. We determined that use of a calcium channel blocker appeared to be detrimental in terms of leg incision outcome. A concurrent study at Bowman Gray Medical Center also found adverse postoperative complications with the use of intravenous calcium channel blockers (Legualt et al., 1996). The Bowman Gray study found that patients receiving this medication were much more likely to have excessive bleeding in the postoperative period. As a result of this finding, their study was terminated early. For our population, we hypothesized that patients who received calcium channel blockers experienced additional bleeding at the leg incision site that led to complications after surgery. Therefore, we have educated our staff about these findings and have curtailed the use of such agents as much as possible at our institution in the postoperative setting.

The most important message to the surgical team at our institution was that this project was able to dispel ideas previously believed to be important to patient outcome. By employing an organized group effort, we were able to identify practice issues that were critical to our patients and to modify our daily practice. The nurses involved in this project realized that, by managing and analyzing data, they could play a leading role in improving patient care.

PLANNING FUTURE PATIENT OUTCOMES PROJECTS

On the basis of our findings, changes have been made in the daily practice at our institution. To determine the impact of these changes on leg incision outcomes, we are currently tracking the incidence of leg wound complications. Evaluation of the changes in practice are critical to continuing improvements in patient care.

REFERENCES

Conklin, C. M., Gray, R. J., Neilson, D., Wong, P., Tomita, D. K., & Matloff, J. M. (1988). Determinants of wound infection incidence after isolated coronary artery bypass surgery in patients randomized to receive prophylactic cefuroxime or cefazolin. *Annals of Thoracic Surgery, 46,* 172-177.

Gentry, L. O., Zeluff, B. J., & Cooley, D. A. (1988). Antibiotic prophylaxis in open-heart surgery: A comparison of cefamandole, cefuroxime, and cefazolin. *Annals of Thoracic Surgery, 46,* 167-171.

Goldsborough, M. A., Miller, M. H., Gibson, J., Creighton-Kelly, S., Custer, C. A., Wallop, J. M., & Greene, P. S. (1999). Incidence of leg wound complications following coronary artery bypass grafting: Identification of risk factors. *American Journal of Critical Care, 8,* 149-153.

Katz, N. M., & Chase, G. A. (1997). Risks of cardiac operations for elderly patients— Reduction of the age factor. *Annals of Thoracic Surgery, 63,* 1309-1314.

Leguält, C., Furberg, C. D., Wagenknecht, L. E., Rogers, A. T., Stump, A. T., & Stump, D. A. (1996). Nimodipine neuroprotection in cardiac valve replacement: Report of an early terminated trial. *Stroke, 27,* 593-598.

McKhann, G. M., Goldsborough, M. A., & Borowicz, L. M. (1997). Predictors of stroke risk in coronary artery bypass patients. *Annals of Thoracic Surgery, 63,* 516-521.

Paradox, Version 8 [Computer software]. (1998). Scotts Valley, CA: Inprise.

Shuhaiber, H., Chugh, T., Portoian-Shuhaiber, S., & Ghosh, D. (1987). Wound infection in cardiac surgery. *Journal of Cardiovascular Surgery, 28,* 139-142.

Townsend, T. R., Reitz, B. A., Bilker, W. B., & Bartlett, J. G. (1993). Clinical trial of cefamandole, cefazolin, and cefuroxime for antibiotic prophylaxis in cardiac operations. *Journal of Thoracic and Cardiovascular Surgery, 106,* 664-670.

Visintainer, M. (1986). Chi square. In B. H. Munro, M. A. Visintainer, & E. B. Page (Eds.), *Statistical methods for health care research* (pp. 127-173). Philadelphia: J. B. Lippincott.

Wells, F. C., Newsom, S. W. B., & Rowlands, C. (1983). Wound infection in cardio-thoracic surgery. *Lancet, 1,* 1209-1210.

CHAPTER 8

Evaluation of the Effect of a Critical Pathway for Patients Undergoing Coronary Artery Bypass Graft

Suzanne J. Rumble

Marinell H. Jernigan

Pamela T. Rudisill

EDITORS' NOTE: Although the use of critical pathways is now widespread, there is little in the literature that describes outcomes associated with these pathways. One of the barriers often sited is the inability of institutional databases to account for patient acuity—for example, by distinguishing patients having their first heart surgery from those having a second or third heart surgery. This chapter describes the arduous work of a graduate nursing student who conducted a manual chart review on 780 cardiac surgery patients to determine whether a care pathway made a difference in length of stay and readmission rate. Her statistical analysis and graphic display of the outcomes data are simple and elegant. This project is sure to inspire the advancement of administrative databases and new alliances between graduate nursing programs and health services agencies seeking assistance in measuring patient outcomes.

IDENTIFYING THE PATIENT OUTCOME

Approximately 57 million Americans have one or more types of cardiovascular disease. Coronary heart disease caused 487,490 deaths in the United States in 1994, and it remains the leading cause of mortality and premature morbidity in the United States. The cost of cardiovascular diseases and stroke in 1997 was estimated to be $259.1 billion. Coronary artery bypass graft (CABG) surgery is a high-cost, high-volume, surgical diagnosis-related group for the treatment of coronary heart disease, with an estimated 501,000 procedures performed on 318,000 patients in 1994. The average cost of coronary artery bypass surgery in 1992 was $44,200 (American Heart Association, 1997).

Increasing health care costs have led health care payers to seek competitive prices from health care providers. Health care providers continually struggle with cost containment and strive to implement models of care delivery that control cost and resource use without compromising the quality of care rendered.

According to Zander (1993), the use of critical pathways is a frequently cited strategy to decrease the fragmentation of services and cost of care. One way to evaluate the effectiveness of critical pathways is to monitor outcomes, such as length of stay, readmission rates, morbidity, mortality, and patient satisfaction (Ebener, Baugh, & Formella, 1996). Rudisill, Phillips, and Payne (1994) examined the use of critical pathways for CABG and heart valve surgery patients at one metropolitan hospital between June and November 1992. The sample consisted of 332 patients. Patient length of stay was decreased by 1.12 days for patients on the critical pathway when compared with patients not on the critical pathway. The average cost per patient decreased by $11,893, resulting in a total institutional savings of $965,487.

Strong and Sneed (1991) studied 28 CABG patients whose care was guided by a critical pathway for a 3-month period at one southeastern medical center. They found that 57% of the patients were discharged within the critical pathway time frame.

Hofmann (1993) evaluated 45 CABG patients: 24 who were cared for without the critical pathway and 20 who received care that included the critical pathway. Study findings revealed that patients on the critical pathway had a decreased length of stay and complication rate when compared with patients not on the pathway. Tidwell (1993) described a multidisciplinary tracking system for use in cardiac surgery case management. This study revealed a decrease in length of stay after the implementation of a CABG critical pathway, and analysis of patient charges showed a 24% reduction for patients following CABG with coronary angiogram.

Readmission rate is another important outcome measure after CABG surgery, but the literature reveals few studies that use readmission as an outcome variable. Hospital readmissions have major implications for health care financing and patient well-being. Anderson and Steinburg (1984) studied randomly selected Medicare beneficiaries who were readmitted after hospital discharge between 1974 and 1977 to examine the proportion of Medicare expenditures attributable to readmissions to the hospital. Their data revealed that 22% of

Medicare hospitalizations were followed by a readmission within 60 days of discharge. Medicare spent more than $2.5 billion per year on readmissions that occurred within 60 days.

In a study by Lubitz, Gornick, Mentneck, and Loop (1993), 53,715 patients who underwent CABG surgery were reviewed from October 1986 through June 1987 using Medicare hospital claims data for readmission rates. The rehospitalization rate after CABG surgery within a year for any reason was 629 per 1,000 live discharges. The average cost of rehospitalization for related events within the year after CABG surgery was $1,207 per patient. The authors concluded that the volume and costs to Medicare for readmissions after CABG surgery make it an important outcome measure.

Stanton and coworkers (1985) examined 326 CABG patients from four medical centers for readmission rates. Interviews and questionnaires that were mailed within the first 6 postoperative months revealed a readmission rate of 24%. The identification and treatment of complications and readmission rates can be important outcome measures of the quality of care delivered (Metcalf, 1991).

As a graduate student at the University of North Carolina at Charlotte, the first author of this chapter (S. R.) was interested in studying the care of patients undergoing cardiovascular surgery. On the basis of a literature review and discussion with the cardiovascular clinical nurse specialist (CNS) at Presbyterian Hospital in Charlotte, North Carolina, she decided to conduct a study to evaluate the effectiveness of critical pathways on the care of patients following CABG surgery. The objective of the study was to provide clinical and financial data associated with pathway use.

BUILDING THE TEAM

The original idea for this project was conceived by the cardiovascular CNS (P. R.), who was a key member of the health care team that developed critical pathways at Presbyterian Hospital and a member of this study team. The graduate student served as the researcher and project leader for the study, which was completed in partial fulfillment of the requirements of a master's degree in nursing. Additional members of the project team included the cardiovascular recovery unit (CVRU) nurse manager, the director for cardiovascular services, and the quality assurance nurse. Team members were selected because of their extensive work with CABG patients prior to and after the implementation of critical pathways.

The Researcher

In addition to being a graduate student, the researcher (S. R.) is a registered nurse and staff member in the CVRU. Discussions with the thesis committee, which included the CNS and nursing professors at the college of nursing, provided the researcher with feedback and approval for the implementation of the study. Institutional support was obtained from the CVRU nurse manager and the director for cardiovascular services, a registered nurse.

The Cardiovascular CNS

The cardiovascular CNS implemented critical pathways for CABG patients at the institution in 1992. She collected data daily from the time critical pathways were implemented at the institution concerning patient outcomes, such as length of stay and adherence to the critical pathway. In addition, she recorded deviations from the critical pathway. The reasons for these deviations were categorized as patient, institution, physician, or nurse.

Multidisciplinary Group

The CNS presented these early data on patient outcomes to the multidisciplinary group that included the CVRU nurse manager, CVRU staff, the surgeons, the respiratory therapist, and the staff on the cardiac step-down unit. This group adopted a collaborative approach that produced major changes in the care of CABG patients in this CVRU in areas such as time to extubation and mobilization. On the basis of a literature review and readmission data, the CNS proposed that readmission rates after CABG surgery be examined to gain one measure of the effectiveness of critical pathways.

Nurse Manager for the CVRU

The CVRU nurse manager worked closely with the CNS and supported the project from the beginning. She assisted the researcher by providing the CVRU log, which contained information about all cardiac surgical patients operated on at the institution.

Quality Assurance Nurse

The researcher met with the quality assurance nurse, who had collected data on readmission rates for all cardiac surgical and medical patients. She determined that approximately 7% of all cardiac surgical patients were readmitted. This information was based on approximately 500 CABG surgeries performed within 1 year and was valuable in planning for the sample size needed to determine whether using critical pathways had influenced readmission rates.

The consulted statistician performed a power analysis and explained that to capture a difference in this small percentage of readmissions, a large sample size was needed. The researcher determined that to examine CABG patients prior to and after the implementation of critical pathways, she would need to use patient data from two different years. All CABG patients who fit the inclusion criteria would be examined for readmission. The years 1991 and 1993 were chosen because these admissions reflected CABG surgeries performed before and after critical pathways, respectively. The year 1992 was omitted because critical pathways were implemented that year, and patients were not consistently placed on the pathway initially. The CVRU log, provided by the nurse manager, included all CABG patients that had surgery. The log contained patients' medical record numbers, ages, gender, procedures, and surgeons. Information about the sample and the plan to obtain these data were presented to the thesis committee. The researcher developed a design for the study and an instrument to collect the data.

SELECTING THE INSTRUMENT

The purpose of this retrospective study was to compare readmission rates for CABG patients who were cared for with and without critical pathways. An instrument that the researcher designed was used to obtain information from selected patients' charts. Data collection included the patient medical record number, age, gender, surgical procedure, name of surgeon, hospital length of stay, surgical length of stay, use of critical pathway, number of readmissions, and readmission diagnosis (Table 8.1). Readmission was defined as any hospital readmission after CABG surgery within 365 days of discharge. Hospital length of stay was defined as day of hospital admission through day of discharge. Surgical length of stay was defined as day of surgery through day of discharge. Inclusion criteria for the sample ($N = 780$) consisted of adult patients who (a) had the surgical procedure performed for the first time by a selected group of cardiovascular surgeons, (b) had no follow-up surgery planned, (c) were hospitalized on one cardiovascular or step-down unit, (d) underwent CABG surgery within 1 year, and (e) were placed on a critical pathway or underwent CABG surgery within 1 year and were not placed on a critical pathway. The patient medical record numbers obtained from the CVRU log were submitted to the medical records department for retrieval and data collection. In support of this project, the medical records department retrieved charts from long lists of patient medical record numbers. The researcher collected all data manually from the charts.

MEASURING THE PATIENT OUTCOME

The time required to obtain data from 780 charts and enter this information into the computer was a major barrier to the conduct of this study. Multiple hours were spent by the researcher obtaining data from the patients' charts that could

TABLE 8.1 Critical Pathway Evaluation Instrument

Medical Record Number	Age	Gender	Surgeon	Hospital LOS	Surgical LOS	Critical Path	Re-Admis.	Re-Admis. Diagnosis

not be removed from the medical records department. The sample ($N = 780$) consisted of 379 patients with CABG surgery whose care did not include use of the critical pathway and 401 CABG patients whose care did include use of the critical pathway. The data were then entered into the computer for analysis by a statistician.

ANALYZING THE DATA

Descriptive statistics were used to provide information about the sample. Percentages were obtained for the dichotomous variables of gender, critical path, and readmission. The interval level variables of age, hospital length of stay, and surgical length of stay were analyzed to obtain means and standard deviations. A t-test analysis was performed to determine whether there was a difference in

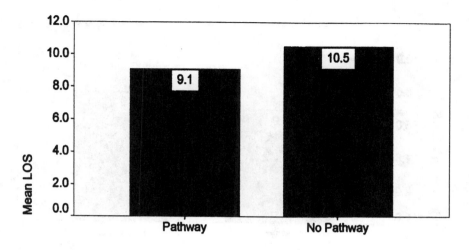

Pathway Status

Figure 8.1. Mean hospital LOS by pathway status ($N = 780$): t test demonstrated a significant difference at p < .05.

length of stay between patients whose care was or was not guided by a critical pathway. A chi-square analysis was used to determine whether an association existed between the variables of critical pathway use and readmission.

SUMMARIZING THE FINDINGS

The sample ($N = 780$) consisted of 379 patients who underwent CABG surgery between January 1, 1991, and December 31, 1991, whose care did not involve use of the critical pathway and 401 patients who underwent CABG surgery between January 1, 1993, and December 31, 1993, whose care did involve use of the critical pathway. The patients included 570 (73%) men and 210 (27%) women, with a mean age of 63.2 years ($SD = 10.7$). The difference in the mean length of stay (LOS) for patients in each group is depicted in Figure 8.1. A t test revealed a significant difference between patients whose care was guided by a critical pathway ($M = 9.1$) and patients whose care was not guided by a pathway ($M = 10.5$, $p = .0001$).

The difference in the mean length of surgical stay for patients in the critical pathway and no critical pathway group is depicted in Figure 8.2. A t test revealed a significant difference between patients whose care was guided by a critical pathway ($M = 6.9$) and patients whose care was not guided by a pathway ($M = 7.9$, $p = .0003$).

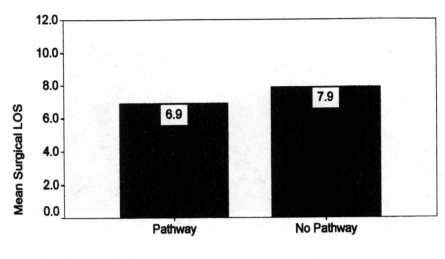

Figure 8.2. Mean surgical LOS by pathway status ($N = 780$): t test demonstrated a significant difference at $p < .05$.

Figure 8.3 reveals the frequency of readmission for patients in the pathway and no pathway groups. A chi-square analysis revealed no significant differences in readmission according to pathway status ($\chi^2 = 0.046$, 1 df, $p = .83$).

APPLYING THE FINDINGS
TO PRACTICE

This study indicates that the use of critical pathways for CABG patients resulted in a decreased hospital LOS and surgical LOS without a significant difference in readmission rates when compared to CABG patients not cared for with the critical pathways. Findings from this study promote critical pathways and a multidisciplinary approach to care.

Critical pathways for CABG patients have facilitated earlier extubation and mobilization. They assist with patient and family education about patient outcomes and caregiver expectations. The nurses document whether a patient adheres to the pathway or deviates from the expected outcome. These findings were presented by the cardiovascular CNS to a joint practice committee consisting of CVRU nurses, surgeons, and nurse managers. After reviewing these data, the cardiovascular CNS began to meet regularly with CABG patients in the sur-

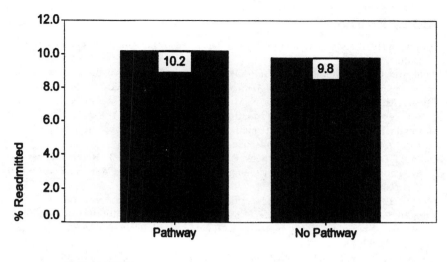

Figure 8.3. Percentage of patients readmitted by pathway status ($N = 780$): Chi-square demonstrated no significant difference.

geon's office following discharge. The patients were examined and complications were documented for further consideration by the health care team.

PLANNING FUTURE PATIENT OUTCOMES PROJECTS

It would be interesting to study the type of patient problems identified by the cardiovascular CNS or nurse practitioner during the postdischarge period and the impact of the nursing interventions on recovery. The finding in this study that critical pathways are associated with a decrease in length of stay without an increase in the readmission rate is exciting. It may be informative, however, to examine the reasons for patient readmission to determine if there are other opportunities for improving care.

This study can serve as a model for health professionals in other specialty areas who wish to examine the effectiveness of critical pathway-guided care. Administrative support is needed to provide the manpower or time needed to obtain data from medical records. Also, collaboration among health care providers was a key factor in the successful completion of this project. Future efforts to develop and use critical pathways should include this team approach.

REFERENCES

American Heart Association. (1997). *1997 heart and stroke statistical update.* Author: Dallas, TX.

Anderson, G. F., & Steinberg, E. P. (1984). Hospital readmissions in the medicare population. *New England Journal of Medicine, 311*(22), 1349-1353.

Ebener, M., Baugh, K., & Formella, N. M. (1996). Proving that less is more: Linking resources to outcome. *Journal of Nursing Care Quality, 10*(2), 1-9.

Hofmann, P. A. (1993). Critical path method: An important tool for coordinating clinical care. *Journal on Quality Improvement, 19*(7), 235-246.

Lubitz, J. D., Gornick, M. E., Mentneck, R. M., & Loop, F. D. (1993). Rehospitalizations after coronary revascularization among Medicare beneficiaries. *American Journal of Cardiology, 72,* 26-30.

Metcalf, E. M. (1991). The orthopedic critical path. *Orthopaedic Nursing, 10*(6), 25-31.

Rudisill, P. T., Phillips, M., & Payne, C. M. (1994). Clinical paths for the cardiac surgery patients: Multidisciplinary approach to QI outcomes. *Journal of Nursing Care Quality, 8*(3), 27-33.

Stanton, A. B., Jenkins, D., Goldstein, R. L., Salm, T. J., Klein, M. D., & Aucoin, R. A. (1985). Hospital readmissions among survivors six months after myocardial revascularization. *Journal of the American Medical Association, 253*(24), 3568-3573.

Strong, A. G., & Sneed, N. V. (1991). Clinical evaluation of a critical path for coronary artery bypass surgery patients. *Progress in Cardiovascular Nursing, 6,* 29-37.

Tidwell, S. L. (1993). A graphic tool for tracking variance & comorbidities in cardiac surgery case management. *Progress in Cardiovascular Nursing, 8*(2), 6-19.

Zander, K. (1993). Toward a fully integrated caremap and case management system. *The New Definition, 8*(2), 25-27.

FURTHER READING

Coffey, R. J., Richards, J. S., Remmert, C. S., Leroy, S. S., Schoville, R. R., & Baldwin, P. J. (1992). An introduction to critical paths. *Quality Management in Health Care, 1,* 45-54.

Cohen, D. J., Breall, J. A., Kalon, K. L., Weintraub, R. M., Kuntz, R. E., Weinstein, M. C., & Baim, D. S. (1993). Economics of elective coronary revascularization: Comparison of costs and charges for conventional angioplasty, directional atherectomy, stenting, and bypass surgery. *Journal of the American College of Cardiology, 22*(4), 1052-1059.

Hamilton, W. M., Hammermeister, K. E., DeRouen, T. A., Zia, M. S., & Dodge, H. T. (1983). Effect of coronary artery bypass grafting on subsequent hospitalization. *American Journal of Cardiology, 51*(3), 353-360.

Hawthorne, M. H. (1994). Gender differences in recovery after coronary artery surgery. *Image: Journal of Nursing Scholarship, 26,* 75-80.

Zander, K. (1987). Critical paths: Marking the course. *Definition, 2*(3), 19-20.

Zander, K. (1989). Second generation critical paths. *Definition, 4*(4), 48-50.

CHAPTER 9

Quality of Life Following the Whipple Procedure

JoAnn Coleman

EDITORS' NOTE: Information technology has enabled patients to take greater control of their health care. When weighing the benefits and burdens of treatment options, patients with serious illness are more frequently asking not only about the length of life but also about the quality of life to be achieved with treatment. Recently, many patients who accessed the Johns Hopkins Medical Institutions' Pancreatic web site contacted JoAnn Coleman, the case manager for pancreas and biliary surgery, to ask what life would be like after the Whipple procedure for pancreatic cancer. Without the necessary time or funding, JoAnn found creative ways to study the outcome of quality of life and provide the answers that people needed.

IDENTIFYING THE PATIENT OUTCOME

Since Whipple, Parsons, and Mullins described the en bloc resection of the head of the pancreas and the duodenum for periampullary malignancies in 1935, surgeons have been challenged to perform one of the most difficult gastrointestinal operations—a pancreaticoduodenectomy. The operation is now referred to as the "Whipple procedure."

The Whipple procedure has been in and out of favor throughout the years. In the 1960s and 1970s, one in every four patients died in the perioperative period. Survival from the operation, and the hospitalization, continued to be grim until the late 1980s (Christ, Sitzmann, & Cameron, 1987). Currently, due to the perseverance of some surgeons and advances in critical care management, the Whipple procedure is an accepted operation for malignant and benign conditions.

127

Examples of malignancies for which the Whipple procedure is performed are tumors of the head of the pancreas, the ampulla, the distal common bile duct, and the duodenum. The most common benign condition is chronic pancreatitis. In the hands of our experienced surgeons at The Johns Hopkins Hospital and those at other hospitals in which a high volume of these procedures are performed, patient mortality and morbidity have reached low levels, with mortality rates of 2% or 3% (Gordon, Burleyson, Tielsch, & Cameron, 1995). What was previously considered a high-risk operation with poor outcomes has become standard surgery for any age group. Most patients are discharged from the hospital within 9 to 12 days postoperatively and today are experiencing the longest survival from this operation than at any previous time. For patients undergoing Whipple procedures for all diagnoses, Yeo et al. (1997) reported 1- and 5-year actuarial survival rates of 79% and 43%, respectively, with a few patients surviving as long as 20 years.

The Whipple procedure is a radical surgical procedure involving the removal of the distal common bile duct; the gallbladder; the head, neck, and uncinate process of the pancreas; the duodenum; and, in some cases, the distal stomach. The gastrointestinal tract is then reconstructed to allow normal digestion. Patients are usually able to resume a normal diet and activity level after initial recovery. Some patients may require insulin therapy after surgery, and all patients receive pancreatic enzymes to assist in fat digestion. Nevertheless, some common complaints by patients after the Whipple procedure are difficulty gaining weight, gastrointestinal symptoms such as diarrhea and early satiety, and nutritional problems. There is concern that these and other conditions may contribute to an unacceptable quality of life after the procedure. This is especially a concern in debilitated older patients. Because these patients have little hope for a curative operation, the quality of life achieved after surgery is a critical outcome.

In my role as case manager for pancreatic and biliary surgery at The Johns Hopkins Hospital, I manage the perioperative care of all patients with pancreatic problems and related surgeries. A research nurse in the department of surgery, who has been involved in studies on patients with pancreatic and biliary disorders, works with me in providing care for these patients. We provide preoperative education, obtain informed consent for research studies, and follow patients through their hospitalization, after discharge, including adjuvent therapies, to the end of life. If patients or referring physicians have questions about the care of patients who undergo the Whipple procedure, we are available by phone to answer them. With the initiation of The Johns Hopkins Medical Institutions (JHMI) pancreas cancer web site that includes our phone number, these calls have increased.

The number of Whipple procedures performed by the Johns Hopkins surgeons annually has steadily increased since 1984 (Figure 9.1). The vast experience of these surgeons, coupled with a multidisciplinary group approach to the

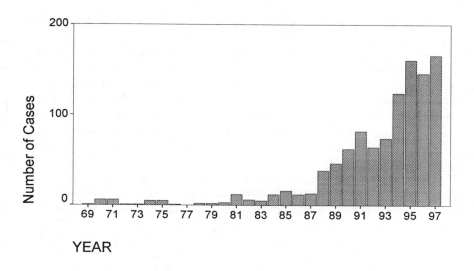

Figure 9.1. Annual Frequency of Pancreaticoduodenectomies at The Johns Hopkins Hospital

treatment of pancreatic cancer, has led to increasingly favorable postoperative patient outcomes. As the length of life increased following the Whipple procedure, we began to consider the impact of this surgery on other patient outcomes. Many patients with whom we spoke had been given misinformation about the procedure, their length of hospital stay, the amount of pain after surgery, and life following recovery from surgery. In an effort to provide accurate information to answer patients' questions about life after the Whipple procedure, the research nurse and I decided to explore quality of life.

QUALITY OF LIFE

Quality of life has gained acceptance in recent years as an important factor when deciding on the appropriate treatment of a disease or condition. For this study, quality of life was defined as a subjective evaluation of the attributes, either positive or negative, that characterize a person's life (Padilla, Ferrell, Grant, & Rhiner, 1990). Health-related quality of life is usually related to the physical, psychological, and social domains of health (Testa & Simonson, 1996). These domains are influenced by experiences, beliefs, expectations, and perceptions. Padilla et al. (1990) discussed the three quality of life domains of psychological, social, and financial functioning. Ferrell, Rhiner, and Rivera (1993) identified the following domains in the quality of life of patients with cancer who were experiencing pain: physical, psychological, social, and spiritual. The physical domain included functional ability, strength and fatigue, sleep and rest, nausea, appetite, and constipation. The psychological domain included anxiety, depression, enjoyment and leisure, pain distress, happiness, fear and cognition, and attention. The social domain included caregiver burden, roles and relationships, affection and sexual function, and appearance. The spiritual domain included suffering, meaning of pain, religiosity, and transcendence. Furthermore, some aspects of quality of life may be associated or correlated with another aspect of quality of life, such as an association between nausea, pain, and fatigue (Piper, 1993).

Very little has been reported on quality of life in patients following the Whipple procedure. Long-term follow-up has been discussed only in terms of survival from surgery as an estimate of quality of life (Lygidakis et al., 1986). Quality of life was mentioned in a study comparing the Whipple procedure with other surgical approaches (Taschiere et al., 1995). The dimension of pain in relation to quality of life was measured in another study that compared the pylorus-preserving Whipple procedure with the duodenum-sparing pancreatic head resection in patients who had chronic pancreatitis (Buchler, Friess, Muller, Wheatley, & Berger, 1995). At the 6-month follow-up examination, 75% of the patients who had the duodenum-sparing surgery were pain free versus 40% who had the pylorus-preserving Whipple. McLeod et al. (1995) measured quality of life, nutritional status, and gastrointestinal hormone profile in patients following the Whipple procedure for either benign or malignant neoplasms compared to patients after a cholecystectomy. The following instruments were used in this study to measure quality of life: the Time Trade-Off Technique instrument, the Direct Questioning of Objectives instrument, the Gastrointestinal Quality of Life Index, the Sickness Impact Profile, and the Physician Global Assessment instrument. Results showed that patients who had the Whipple procedure and remained disease-free reported high levels of quality of life.

Finally, Melvin et al. (1998) examined the postoperative nutritional status, pancreatic exocrine and endocrine function, and subjective quality of life parameters in 45 patients having either a standard Whipple procedure or a pylorus-preserving Whipple procedure. The Short Form-36 health survey was used to measure quality of life. There were few early or late differences seen between the two groups, indicating a positive postoperative quality of life and normal nutritional parameters in most patients regardless of the type of procedure performed.

Quality of life is an important factor for patients undergoing extensive surgery such as the Whipple procedure. With the exception of the studies previously mentioned, however, few studies have addressed quality of life. Some studies used no quality of life tool, examining only survival as a measure of quality of life, or the surgeon's perception of the patient's quality of life. When quality of life was assessed, many different tools were used because quality of life represents many domains. This has made it difficult to compare study results. Because of the small number of studies examining exclusively the patient's perspective, we decided to explore the effect of the Whipple procedure on quality of life from the patient's perspective.

BUILDING THE TEAM

Initially, the research team consisted of the Department of Surgery research nurse and myself. We discussed our idea for a quality of life study with the attending surgeons who perform the Whipple procedure, and we found that we could add our quality of life instrument to an existing research protocol in which patients had consented to survey follow-up after discharge. Later, a medical student also joined our team.

SELECTING AN INSTRUMENT

We had been in a quandary about an instrument to evaluate quality of life in these patients. Many instruments were reviewed, but none met our mutual requirement that the survey be short, simple, and self-administered. I happened to attend an American Cancer Society nursing research conference and was pleasantly surprised to be given the quality of life instrument we eventually selected in a packet of information supplied to all in attendance.

The Quality of Life Tool (patient version) developed by Ferrell and Rhiner at the City of Hope National Medical Center, Duarte, California (Appendix A), was selected to assess patients' quality of life after a Whipple procedure (Ferrell, Dow, & Grant, 1995). This 30-item linear analog scale contains a 10-cm line for each item with an anchor at each end indicating a positive or negative aspect of quality of life. The patient is asked to place an "X" on the line to indicate what is currently happening regarding that item. The instrument can be self-administered and is relatively brief and easy to complete. In addition, the tool has been tested with established reliability (test-retest and internal consistency) and validity (content, construct, and concurrent). It has been used to test quality of life in many patients with cancer, including cancer survivors and patients with a disease-specific cancer (Dow, Ferrell, Leigh, Ly, & Gulasekaram, 1996; Ferrell et al., 1995; Grant et al., 1992).

To score each item on the Quality of Life Tool, a 10-cm ruler is placed at the far left-hand edge of the line with the 0 placed at the very edge of the line. The distance is measured from 0 to the point where the patient has placed the X. That number is placed in the margin on the right-hand side of the tool for data entry. In most cases, higher scores indicate greater quality of life. Several items have reverse anchors, and therefore the number obtained is subtracted from

10 and placed in the right-hand margin for data entry. The 30 questions can be broken down into three domains. Fifteen questions measure physical aspects of quality of life, 5 questions relate to the social domain, and 10 questions assess the psychosocial domain.

MEASURING THE PATIENT OUTCOME

A large database is kept on each patient having a Whipple procedure at The Johns Hopkins Hospital for many reasons, particularly for research aimed at improving the care of patients having this procedure. Therefore, the names and addresses were readily available. A special "tickler file" was prepared for reminding us to attend to matters at a future date. Questionnaires, along with self-addressed, stamped envelopes, were initially sent to all patients at 1 month and then every 3 months after surgery. We later realized that this mailing schedule was too frequent because replies from the patients indicated that little had changed since the last measurement period. We then decided to send out questionnaires at 6-month intervals after surgery. The result was a better picture of how patients rated their quality of life because most patients had just completed a 6-month course of adjuvant chemoradiation therapy. The returned questionnaires provided a wealth of information about how patients perceive their health after their surgery, including those who also had adjuvant therapy. Many patients wrote notes to us, and family members returned questionnaires with information of a patient's death, even describing the patient's quality of life during the terminal period. Thus, our measurement of quality of life provided us with length of survival and insight into patients' last days of life.

Two hundred and eighty questionnaires were collected during a 2-year period. As the number of patients undergoing Whipple procedure and participating in research studies increased, we stopped mailing the quality of life questionnaires due to lack of time. Changes in funding also hampered our ability to obtain stamps and stationary. The questionnaires were stacked in a cabinet with good intentions of analyzing the data at some time in the future. Not until I had the good fortune to have a graduate nursing student spend a semester learning about case management with a major emphasis on measuring patient outcomes did we have an opportunity to analyze the data. The student was eager to provide the important service of creating a database and entering and analyzing patient responses on the linear analog scale. Because she was also fulfilling her course objectives, we all benefited from her involvement. The scores were entered using the statistical program SPSS (1994). Frequencies of responses for each question were determined, along with the mean, mode, and standard deviation for each item and the entire instrument. Correlations were examined between selected questions using the Pearson's product moment (r) correlation coefficient.

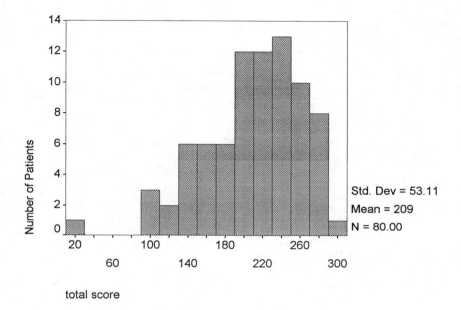

Figure 9.2. Quality of Life in Patients 6 Months After Whipple Procedure

ANALYZING THE DATA

Six-Month Outcomes

Of the 280 completed surveys, the graduate student was able to enter data from 80 during her semester of work. These 80 surveys were from an initial mailing within 6 months after surgery. The frequency distribution of total scores is illustrated in a histogram (Figure 9.2). The range of total scores was 11 to 300, with a mean of 209 (*SD* = 53.11).

Means were calculated for each question. There was a potential item range of 0 to 10, and all items were transposed for analysis so that 0 equaled the worst outcome and 10 equaled the best outcome. The lowest mean item score was 4.61 for the question "Do you tire easily?" This indicates that fatigue is a problem for many patients. The highest mean score was for the question about the subject's ability to move around inside the hospital room or home. With the exception of the question about fatigue, all mean scores were higher than the midpoint of 5.0, indicating a good of quality of life.

Correlations were performed between the question "How good is your quality of life?" and selected questions measuring levels of fatigue, control, pain,

TABLE 9.1 Correlation Between Quality of Life Question and Selected Other
Questions ($N = 80$)

How good is your quality of life?	Pearson's Correlation Coefficient	p Value
Do you tire easily?	−.51	.001
Do you feel like you are in control of things in your life?	.51	.001
Do you have nausea?	−.42	.001
How much pain do you have?	−.35	.002
How much of an appetite do you have?	.30	.008
Is the support you receive from others sufficient to meet your needs?	.25	.031

appetite, nausea, and social support (Table 9.1). As previously stated, the presence of fatigue or tiredness, pain, and nausea have previously been negatively correlated to quality of life (Piper, 1993). The same correlations were present in this study. In all cases, there was a weak to moderate correlation when comparing fatigue, pain, appetite, nausea, and social support with the patients' assessment of their quality of life.

Two-Year Outcomes

The graduate nursing student's final paper and presentation of her preliminary findings from 80 patients revealed a favorable quality of life in patients after a Whipple procedure. This information was then presented to one of the surgeons because the question of quality of life after pancreatic surgery had just been debated at a weekly gastrointestinal surgery conference. The surgeon was completely surprised at the amount of information collected, the preliminary favorable findings, and the statistical significance. On learning that there were even more data to be analyzed, he insisted that this be a priority endeavor. Although the research nurse and I agreed with the surgeon regarding the importance of this project, we did not have time to enter and analyze the data given our existing commitments. I explained to the surgeon that if he could find a medical student interested in providing data support for the project, I would be happy to

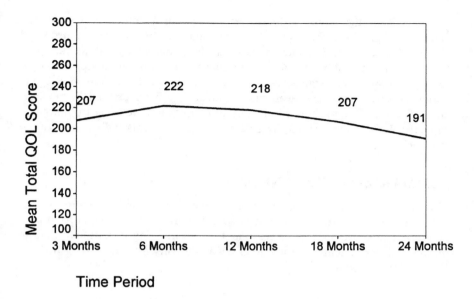

Figure 9.3. Quality of Life Changes Over Time (N = 187; Potential Range, 0-300; Higher Scores Indicate Greater Quality of Life)

continue the project. The next day, a medical student knocked on my door and volunteered to enter the rest of the data and perform the final analysis. Because of the medical student's interest, time, and computer abilities, he was able to complete these tasks promptly. Recently, the surgical department acquired additional funding for pancreatic cancer that has enabled us to resurrect the mailing of questionnaires via a computerized system with clerical support. This project has become an important tool for the surgeons, myself, and the research nurse to use in answering patients' and others' questions about what to expect after surgery and, in particular, what quality of life to expect after recovery from the procedure.

With the assistance of the medical student, 200 returned questionnaires were examined, of which 187 were appropriate or acceptable for data analysis. Using Microsoft Excel (1997), the medical student entered and analyzed the data by months at 3, 6, 12, 18, and 24 months from time of surgery. Figure 9.3 depicts changes in quality of life from 3 to 24 months after surgery. Patients rated higher than the midpoint of the quality of life instrument at all five time periods. An improvement in quality of life was seen at 6 and 12 months after the Whipple procedure, with a slow decline noted at 18 and 24 months. This decline in quality of life may be related to recurrence of cancer.

Analysis of the physical domain subscale scores demonstrated that the patients had good performance at 6 months and even better performance at 12 months. Patients' social achievement subscale scores were good during the 6- to 12-month interval and then very gradually declined. Patients psychologic subscale scores were stable for 12 months followed by a gradual decline. Patients need to be assessed in all three domains to fully understand their experience after the Whipple procedure. The three questions relating to "fatigue," "appetite," and "worry about disease" were areas patients indicated were the most problematic.

SUMMARIZING THE FINDINGS

This study addressed the impact of the Whipple procedure on quality of life. Although problems such as loss of appetite, poor nutrition, fatigue, and pain continue to require aggressive treatment, it is satisfying to note that despite these problems patients continue to enjoy a relatively good quality of life following this procedure.

APPLYING THE FINDINGS TO PRACTICE

Quality of life has become an important priority in health care. Definitions of quality of life have included subjective and objective indicators of both physical and psychological phenomena. Objective indicators, such as income, housing, and physical function, are commonly used as measures of quality of life. These objective indicators, however, do not tell us how individuals perceive their lives. Objective factors are at best only fair indicators of an individual's perceived quality of life. Subjective evaluations define more precisely the experience of life. Therefore, the concept of subjectively perceived quality of life requires analysis as a discrete entity.

In patients with gastrointestinal malignancies, quality of life assessments may be used to aid in the selection of treatments for patients, monitor the quality of care, and direct policy development and resource allocation. The development of new techniques in the diagnosis and treatment of these cancers calls for continued and rigorous evaluation of outcomes. Valid and reliable quality of life measures will provide information about the impact of treatments on quality of life. From the patient's point of view, quality of life considerations may be of paramount importance in making treatment decisions. Quality of life measures may also play an increasingly important role in assessing the benefit of surgical procedures for patients. It is possible that changes in therapy will be developed for the expressed purpose of improving quality of life without any improvement in survival rates. Such procedures will need to be compared with conventional techniques to establish their value.

PLANNING FUTURE PATIENT OUTCOMES PROJECTS

It would be useful to compare the survival and quality of life of patients who do not have the Whipple procedure with those of patients who have had the Whipple procedure. Patients who have the Whipple procedure may be different from patients who choose not to have the procedure. The two groups could be compared on selected variables, such as extent of disease, functional health, hope, and locus of control.

These data could be further divided into subgroup analysis. Because the Whipple operation is performed for malignant and benign disease, these two groups need to be compared. Analysis could be done by types of cancer, including pancreatic, bile duct, and duodenal cancers. Analysis of benign diseases, including chronic pancreatitis and pancreatic cysts, could also be undertaken.

We should study the impact of adjuvant therapy for malignant disease on quality of life. The most prevalent problems identified were fatigue and loss of appetite. Interventions to treat these problems must be tested in this patient population. Prompt follow-up is important to identify and treat these problems early. The issue of age could be analyzed to determine if there is any difference in quality of life in older patients (70 years and older) after the Whipple procedure compared to that of younger patients (younger than 70 years of age) because age is no longer a contraindication to the procedure (Sohn et al., 1998).

These quality outcomes can be used for the education of patients within the institution and beyond. For example, results could be placed on the JHMI pancreatic cancer web site. In addition, quality of life outcomes can be provided to managed care companies when negotiating contracts. Greater efforts continue to be directed at studying the effects of pancreatic disease and its treatment on quality of life. Exercise programs for patients to improve muscle strength and endurance to prevent fatigue could be evaluated in the postoperative and recovery period. Nursing care can then be directed to help patients achieve the best possible outcomes.

REFERENCES

Buchler, M. W., Friess, H., Muller, M. W., Wheatley, A. M., & Berger, H. G. (1995). Randomized trial of duodenum-preserving pancreatic head resection versus pylorus-preserving Whipple in chronic pancreatitis. *American Journal of Surgery, 169,* 65-69.

Christ, D. W., Sitzmann, J. V., & Cameron, J. L. (1987). Improved hospital morbidity, mortality, and survival after the Whipple procedure. *Annals of Surgery, 206*(3), 358-365.

Dow, K. H., Ferrell, B. R., Leigh, S., Ly, J., & Gulasekaram, P. (1996). An evaluation of the quality of life among long-term survivors of breast cancer. *Breast Cancer Research and Treatment, 39,* 261-273.

Excel Version 97 for Windows [Computer software]. (1997). Redmond, WA: Microsoft.

Ferrell, B., Rhiner, M. M., & Rivera, L. M. (1993). Development and evaluation of the family pain questionnaire. *Journal of Psychosocial Oncology, 10*(4), 21-35.

Ferrell, B. R., Dow, K. H., & Grant, M. (1995). Measurement of the quality of life in cancer survivors. *Quality of Life Research, 4,* 523-531.

Gordon, T. A., Burleyson, G. P., Tielsch, J. M., & Cameron, J. L. (1995). The effects of regionalization on cost and outcome for one general high-risk surgical procedure. *Annals of Surgery, 221,* 43-49.

Grant, M., Ferrell, B., Schmidt, G. M., Fonbuena, P., Niland, J. C., & Forman, S. J. (1992). Measurement of quality of life in bone marrow transplantation survivors. *Quality of Life Research, 1,* 375-384.

Lygidakis, N. J., Brummelkamp, W. H., Tytgat, G. H., Huibtegtse, K. H., Lubbers, M. J., van der Meer, A. D., Schenk, K. E., van Gulik, T. M., & Roesing, H. (1986). Periampullary and pancreatic head carcinoma: Facts and factors influencing mortality, survival, and quality of postoperative life. *American Journal of Gastroenterology, 81*(10), 968-974.

McLeod, R. S., Taylor, B. R., O'Connor, B. I., Greenberg, G. R., Jeejeeboy, K. N., Royall, D., & Langer, B. (1995). Quality of life, nutritional status, and gastrointestinal hormone profile following the Whipple procedure. *American Journal of Surgery, 169,* 179-185.

Melvin, W. S., Buekers, K. S., Muscarella, P., Johnson, J. A., Schirmer, W. J., & Ellison, E. C. (1998). Outcome analysis of long-term survivors following pancreaticduodenectomy. *Journal of Gastrointestinal Surgery, 2,* 72-78.

Padilla, G. V., Ferrell, B., Grant, M. M., & Rhiner, M. (1990). Defining the content domain of quality of life for cancer patients with pain. *Cancer Nursing, 13*(2), 108-115.

Piper, B. (1993) Fatigue. In V. Carrieri-Kohlman, A. M. Lindsey, & C. M. West (Eds.), *Pathophysiological phenomena in nursing: Human responses to illness* (2nd ed., pp. 279-301). Philadelphia: W. B. Saunders.

Sohn, T. A., Yeo, C. J., Cameron, J. L., Talamini, M. A., Hruban, R. H., Sauter, P. A., Coleman, J., Ord, S. E., Grochow, L. B., Abrams, R. A., & Pitt, H. A. (1998). Should pancreaticoduodenectomy be performed in octogenarians? *Journal of Gastrointestinal Surgery, 2,* 207-216.

SPSS Version 6.1 for Windows [Computer software]. (1994). Chicago: SPSS.

Taschiere, A. M., Elli, M., Rovati, M., Porretta, T., Montecomozzo, G., Gerlinzani, S., & Cristaldi, M. (1995). Carcinoma of the head of the pancreas: Review of 67 cases and comparison with 27 additional periampullary carcinomas. *Hepato-Gastroenterology, 42*(6), 1023-1025.

Testa, M. A., & Simonson, D. C. (1996). Assessment of quality-of-life outcomes. *Current Concepts, 334*(13), 835-840.

Whipple, A. O., Parsons, W. B., & Mullins, C. R. (1935). Treatment of carcinoma of the ampulla of Vater. *Annals of Surgery, 102,* 763-779.

Yeo, C. J., Cameron, J. L., Sohn, T. A., Lillemoe, K. D., Pitt, H. A., Talamini, M. A., Hruban, R. H., Ord, S. E., Sauter, P. K., Coleman, J. A., Zahurak, M. L., Grochow, L. B., & Abrams, R. A. (1997). Six hundred fifty consecutive pancreaticoduodenectomies in the 1990s, pathology, complications, and outcomes. *Annals of Surgery, 226*(3), 248-260.

The Quality of Life Tool (Patient Version)

Below are a number of questions pertaining to your well-being. Please make an X on the line to indicate what is happening to you at the present. The term "normal for me" means what was normal *prior to illness.*

Below is an example which may help you in responding to the questionnaire.

How do you feel about your ability to concentrate?

Cannot concentrate   Can concentrate
at all _____ X _____ extremely well

   The "X" on the line indicates you are able to concentrate but not 100%.

1. How easy or difficult is it to adjust to your disease and treatment?
Not at all_____ Very easy

2. How much enjoyment are you getting out of life?
None _____ A great deal

3. Do you worry about the cost of your medical care?
Not at all _____ A great deal

4. If you have pain, how distressing is it?

Not at all   Extremely
distressing _____ distressing

5. How useful do you feel?

Not at all   Extremely
useful_____ useful

6. How much happiness do you feel?

None at all _____ A great deal

7. How satisfying is your life?

Not at all   Extremely
satisfying _____ satisfying

8. Is the amount of affection you give and receive sufficient to meet your needs?

Not at all _____ Completely

9. Is your disease or treatment interfering with your personal relationships?

Not at all_____ A great deal

10. Are you worried (fearful or anxious) about the outcome of your disease?

Not at all _____ Constantly

11. How often are you able to do the things you like to do, such as watch
    TV, read, garden, listen to music, etc.?

Not at all_____ A great deal

12. How is your present ability to pay attention to what's happening?

Extremely poor _____ Excellent

13. How much strength do you have?

None at all _____ A great deal

14. Do you tire easily?

Not at all_____ A great deal

15. Is the amount of time you sleep sufficient to meet your needs?

Not at all _____ Completely

16. How good is your quality of life?

Extremely poor _____ Excellent

17. Are you able to take care of your personal needs (dress, hair, toilet, baths, etc.)?

I can't do anything   I can do everything
by myself _____ by myself

18. How much pain do you have?

None _____ A great deal

19. How much of an appetite do you have?

None _____ More than usual

20. How is your bowel pattern?

The worst
I've ever had _____ Normal for me

21. Is the amount you eat sufficient to meet your needs?

Not at all _____ Completely

22. Are you worried about your weight?

Not at all _____ A great deal

23. Do you have nausea?

Never _____ All the time

24. Do you vomit?

Never _____ All the time

25. Have you had any changes in taste?

None at all _____ A great deal

26. Are you able to get around inside your hospital room or home?

Completely   Can get around
bed bound _____ on my own

27. How satisfied are you with your appearance?

Completely   Completely
dissatisfied _____ satisfied

28. Are you worried about unfinished business?

Not at all _____ Extremely

29. Is the support you receive from others sufficient to meet your needs?

Not at all   Completely
sufficient _____ sufficient

30. Do you feel like you are in control of things, of your life?

I feel totally   I feel totally
in control _____ out of control

Developed by B. Ferrell and M. M. Rhiner, City of Hope National Medical Center, Duarte, California

CHAPTER 10

Precursors of Patient Seclusion in a Psychiatric Patient Population

Donna L. Brannan

Judith M. Rohde

EDITORS' NOTE: This chapter provides an excellent example of how a performance improvement approach can be used to examine patient outcomes and improve care. Seeking to minimize the need for placing psychiatric patients in seclusion, this multidisciplinary group examined every aspect of the seclusion process. All seclusion events during an 18-month period were studied. Variables concerning the patients' diagnoses, medical histories, and current health status were examined, as were variables concerning medical and nursing interventions just prior to the seclusion event. Finally, staff and patient injuries during the seclusion process were also recorded. Findings are summarized succinctly, using tables and bar graphs.

IDENTIFYING THE PATIENT OUTCOME

Seclusion is a form of involuntary containment in which an acutely ill psychiatric patient is confined in a room, locked or unlocked. It is indicated for patients whose behavior is dangerous to themselves or others and cannot be managed by any other less restrictive means. The status of the seclusion room as locked or unlocked depends on patients' ability to control their behavior.

Because of its potential untoward effects, the seclusion intervention is closely monitored by psychiatric institutions. Used indiscriminately, seclusion can negatively influence patients' feelings about treatment, expose them to self-

143

injury, and disrupt relationships between the patient and family and the treatment team. The literature on seclusion reflects a common concern about the use of seclusion and its potential for patient neglect and misuse (Angold, 1989; Mason, 1993; Muir-Cochrane, 1996; Richmond, Trujillo, Schmelzer, Phillips, & Davis, 1996; Soloff, Gutheil, & Wexler, 1985; Visalli, McNasser, Johnstone, & Lazzaro, 1997). Another reason that institutions monitor seclusion is to comply with regulatory requirements. The Joint Commission on Accreditation of Health Care Organizations (JCAHO) has assigned the use of this intervention to the category of special treatment procedures with stringent guidelines for clinical justification and documentation. A final reason for monitoring seclusion is its cost. Psychiatric hospitals are confronted with burgeoning clinical acuity, decreasing lengths of stay, and diminishing third-party reimbursement sources. Health care professionals are challenged with caring for patients during the most acute phases of illness, often characterized by patient aggression and violence. It is likely that the frequency of restrictive interventions, such as seclusion, will increase. Along with the prescription of seclusion is the requirement that specific numbers and types of personnel support this practice. These human resource requirements have financial implications for acute care facilities at a time when health care resources are increasingly restricted.

The Department of Psychiatry at The Johns Hopkins Hospital has had a long history of a comprehensive, multidisciplinary approach to clinical performance improvement. High risk and high volume treatments, such as seclusion for psychiatric patients, have long been a priority in the department's performance improvement efforts. When this project began, we believed that if certain patient characteristics and behaviors could be identified as precursors to seclusion, alternative interventions could begin early and the need for seclusion could be minimized. We also thought that a description of interventions prior to seclusion could provide information about current efforts to minimize this treatment. In this first phase of the project, we described the frequency of drug abuse history and violence history among patients placed in seclusion. We also described patient behaviors and staff interventions preceding seclusion.

BUILDING THE TEAM

Psychiatric nursing leaders and frontline direct care providers participated in conceptualizing a performance improvement approach to the analysis of seclusion. Once committed to the decision to monitor seclusion events, the data collection instrument was developed by the Psychiatry Nursing Continuous Quality Improvement Committee. This forum consists of clinical nurse representatives from each inpatient psychiatric unit and the day hospital. The group was selected because the participants are care providers who directly implement this treatment intervention.

The instrument draft underwent periodic review and revision through the multidisciplinary performance improvement team in the department of psychiatry. Although nurses and physicians were the primary participants in tool revisions, the law office and the security department also contributed to development of this indicator. The effort to develop seclusion as a quality performance measure actualized the departmental philosophy that quality activities should have the contribution of as many disciplines as possible. This initiative also encouraged stakeholders to contribute to the monitoring of this high-risk process of care.

The development of this performance measure involved biweekly meetings of the nursing performance improvement representatives. The group discussed fundamental conceptual issues using the hospital performance improvement templates as a guide for measure development. This process included establishing definitions, reviewing the literature, and reviewing regulatory requirements including the JCAHO cycle of performance improvement. The nursing committee forwarded drafts to the departmental performance improvement committee for collaborative review and final approval.

The nursing performance improvement representatives were responsible for coordinating the data collection effort. Each event of seclusion requires the care provider to complete a data collection tool. Thus, individuals directly involved in patient care participated in performance improvement.

SELECTING AN INSTRUMENT

Review of the literature revealed no instrument to record the seclusion variables that represented the characteristics of the patient population and the practice standards in our institution. Historically, the department tracked seclusion events by means of a simple log specifying patient name, time and date seclusion commenced, and time and date seclusion concluded. Staff compliance was poor in completing this log.

On the basis of the experiences of the psychiatric treatment team, the Seclusion Indicator Log (Appendix A) was tailored to our patient population and setting. Each seclusion event was to be documented on this form. The development team members believed that a concise instrument would most likely ensure compliance, and that it would be easily reviewable by state and other regulatory agencies. The data collection instrument included demographic patient information, patient behaviors prior to seclusion, preseclusion staff interventions, PRN psychotropic medication use, and information about possible injuries.

Staff education inservices for all shifts and nurse manager reinforcement of the importance of the analysis of seclusion resulted in a 100% compliance with seclusion performance improvement monitoring. One of the staff's rewards for thorough and complete data collection was the assurance that the data analysis would produce useful information that would be used to improve practice.

We monitored and aggregated total seclusion events in a rate-based method of events per patient day. Some variables were summarized as frequencies in tables or graphs.

MEASURING THE PATIENT OUTCOME

For this phase of the project, we examined seclusion data for an 18-month period from 1995 to 1997. There were 227 patient seclusion events during this reporting period.

The steps in the outcomes measurement process included:

- Unit data collection

- Nurse manager event review

- SPSS software data entry and analysis

- Data review by the Psychiatry Nursing Quality Improvement Committee and the Psychiatric Nursing Leadership Group

- Review by the multidisciplinary Psychiatry Performance Improvement Team

One of the challenges in designing this process was the temptation to overprocess and become bogged down in the details of creating a data collection instrument. It was critical to assign a concise time line so that staff involved would be familiar with the issues as the project advanced. Additional challenges included

- Creating a clear, concise data collection tool

- Identifying essential data components that have potential for improving practice

- Investing time in data collection, entry, and analysis

- Managing the expenses of selection and purchase of a computer system and software capable of running the statistical program

- Consulting with other colleagues about obtaining more advanced methods of analysis

TABLE 10.1 Demographic Data (*N* = 227)

Variable	%
Age	
13-25	23.9
26-50	59.2
51-76	16.9
Psychiatric diagnosis[a]	
Bipolar mania	65.5
Schizophrenia	40.8
Depression	23.1
Dementia	17.6

a. Some patients had two or more diagnoses.

ANALYZING THE DATA

Seclusion variables were expressed as frequencies and seclusion event rate per patient days. At this point, the performance improvement team can generate more sophisticated research questions.

SUMMARIZING THE FINDINGS

Patient demographic data are described in Table 10.1. The variables describing the type of seclusion event and resultant injuries to patients and staff are identified in Table 10.2. These data confirmed our belief that injuries are minimal to staff and patients. We found that of the seclusion events reported, 48% were patients with a substance abuse history (Figure 10.1), and 58% of the patients had a history of violence (Figure 10.2).

The unit breakdown of these patients supported our belief that two of our units maintain the highest proportion of patients with violence and substance abuse history. All the patients secluded exhibited aggressive or nondirectable behavior or both toward self or others (Figure 10.3).

The findings identified areas of strength and areas for performance improvement. We found that staff consistently implemented appropriate preventative interventions in the preseclusion phase (Figure 10.4).

Findings also identified that PRN psychotropic medication administration was frequently and appropriately employed. Selective use of PRN medications

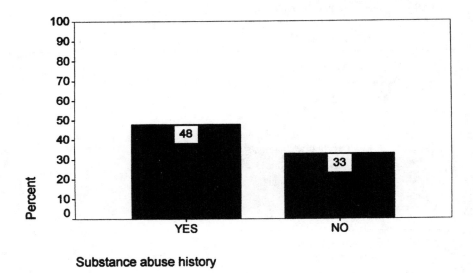

Figure 10.1. Patient History of Substance Abuse, 1995 Through 1997 ($N = 227$)

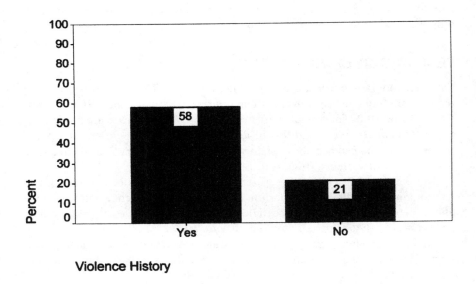

Figure 10.2. Patient History of Violence, 1995 Through 1997 ($N = 227$)

TABLE 10.2 Seclusion Event Type and Outcome Injuries to Patient and Staff

Variable	%
Seclusion event type ($N = 211$)[a]	
Open-door seclusion	30.8
Locked-door seclusion	58.6
Open-door to locked-door seclusion	3.5
Outcome injuries ($N = 227$)	
Patient—Class II (a small scrape, abrasion, or bruise that heals without treatment in a few days)	1.3
Staff—Class II	2.7

a. Does not equal 100% due to missing data.

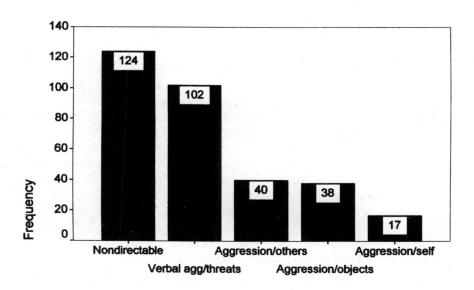

Figure 10.3. Behaviors Precipitating Seclusion, 1995 Through 1997 ($N = 227$)

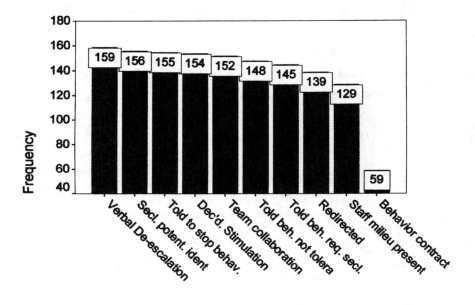

Figure 10.4. Interventions Prior to Seclusion, 1995 Through 1997 ($N = 227$)

is part of accepted practice at our institution to assist in calming a patient with
agitated behavior. Direct care providers in acute psychiatric settings frequently
face the dilemma of how to respect the patient's treatment refusal rights while
promoting the therapeutic use of PRN psychotropic medications that will support the patient's engagement in the treatment process. In a study representing
2,150 seclusion or restraint orders at New York State psychiatric facilities,
56% of the orders were accompanied by a PRN psychotropic medication (Way,
1986). Although it is our practice to use PRNs within the constraints of law
and regulatory requirements, the seclusion performance measure affords the
team an added degree of vigilance in monitoring this practice. In the vast majority of seclusion events, the data demonstrate that nurses considered the option of
administering PRN medications (Figure 10.5).

APPLYING THE FINDINGS TO PRACTICE

The data confirmed our belief that nurses recognize volatile, agitated patients
on the unit and institute deescalating interventions. More than half of our se-

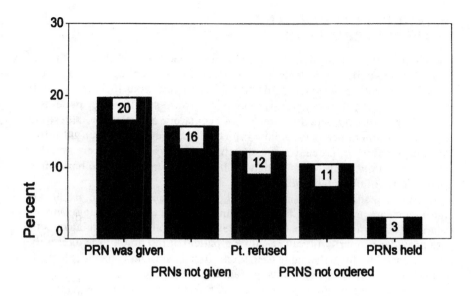

Figure 10.5. PRN Medication Prior to Seclusion, 1995 Through 1997 (*N* = 227)

cluded patient population had substance abuse or violence histories. The findings also suggest that although nurses employed appropriate interventions to prevent seclusion, some seclusion episodes appeared to be unavoidable. We continue to educate nurses about the use of deescalating interventions including PRN medications and the need for multidisciplinary discussions about patient seclusion predictors.

We believe that the low number of patient and staff injuries while initiating and during the seclusion process is due to comprehensive education of all staff in managing patient aggression. The Psychiatric Nursing Aggressive Patient Management Committee is an active workgroup that oversees staff education and safety systems to manage aggressive patients.

On the basis of these findings, we determined that the Aggressive Patient Management Committee and Psychiatric Nursing Continuous Quality Improvement Committee need to combine efforts to develop a measurement tool that addresses many different aspects of aggressive patient management. Working together to collect and review the data will promote performance improvement opportunities and education of staff in patient seclusion predictors and prevention interventions.

PLANNING FUTURE PATIENT
OUTCOMES PROJECTS

The Aggressive Patient Management Committee and the Psychiatric Nursing Continuous Quality Improvement Committee are working together to supplement our current measurement tool with additional questions focused on identifying patients at risk for aggressive behavior toward staff or other patients or both. Given the heightened awareness of regulatory agencies about restraint use, the instrument needs to include information about restraints of all forms. We are planning, as a department, to refine the current method for trending seclusion and restraint events so that we have comparative data to benchmark against those of other facilities.

Our organization has recently undergone reengineering, which produced a significant care provider and skill mix change in our acute care setting. Our new data collection measurement tool will also include information related to the care provider primarily involved with the patient at the time of the aggressive patient episode. This will enable us to track whether skill mix change affects the number and severity of aggressive patient events.

With continued reeducation of staff and refinement of data collection measures, it is our goal to significantly decrease the number of aggressive patient incidents and seclusion and restraint events.

REFERENCES

Angold, A. (1989). Seclusion. *British Journal of Psychiatry, 154,* 437-444.

Mason, T. (1993). Seclusion theory reviewed—A benevolent or malevolent intervention? *Medical Science Law, 33,* 95-102.

Muir-Cochrane, E. (1996). An investigation into nurses' perceptions of secluding patients on closed psychiatric wards. *Journal of Advanced Nursing, 23,* 555-563.

Richmond, I., Trujillo, D., Schmelzer, J., Phillips, S., & Davis, D. (1996). Least restrictive alternatives: Do they really work? *Journal of Nursing Care Quality, 11,* 29-37.

Soloff, P., Gutheil, T., & Wexler, D. (1985). Seclusion and restraint in 1985: A review and update. *Hospital and Community Psychiatry, 36,* 652-657.

Visalli, H., McNasser, G., Johnstone, L., & Lazzaro, C. A. (1997). Reducing high-risk interventions for managing aggression in psychiatric settings. *Journal of Nursing Care Quality, 11,* 54-61.

Way, B. B. (1986). The use of restraint and seclusion in New York State psychiatric centers. *International Journal of Law & Psychiatry, 8,* 383-393.

THE JOHNS HOPKINS HOSPITAL DEPARTMENT OF PSYCHIATRIC NURSING
SECLUSION INDICATOR LOG

Appendix 1

Definition: Involuntary seclusion of a patient whose behavior is dangerous to self or others and cannot be managed by any other less restrictive means.

Patient Name/Age:
 	
History No:
 	
History of substance abuse: (Circle one)
  1) Yes   2) No
History of violence: (Circle one)
  1) Yes   2) No
ED Admission date/time:_____
  1) Yes   2) No
Type of seclusion: (Circle one)
1) Open Door   2) Locked Door   3) Open Door to Locked Door
	Psychiatric Diagnosis: (Circle all that apply)
	
	  1) Bipolar/mania
	  2) Schizophrenia
	  3) Organic Mood Disorder
	  4) Depression
	  5) Dementia
	  6) Personality Disorder
	  7) Substance abuse
	  8) Delirium
	  9) Other _____

Date/Time In:
 	
Date/Time Out:
	Unstable Medical Conditions
	  1) Hepatitis 3) None
	  2) AIDS 4) Other _____

UNIT: 1) MEYER 3
 	
          2) INTENSIVE TREATMENT UNIT
 	
          3) MEYER 4
 	
          4) MEYER 5
 	
          5) MEYER 6
	PRECIPITATING EVENT: (Circle one response for each)
	
	  1) Verbal aggression/threats 1) Yes 2) No
	  2) Physical aggression against objects 1) Yes 2) No
	  3) Physical aggression against self 1) Yes 2) No
	  4) Physical aggression against others 1) Yes 2) No
	  5) Seclusion admission from the ED 1) Yes 2) No
	  6) Nondirectable behavior 1) Yes 2) No
	  7) Other

INTERVENTIONS ATTEMPTED PRIOR TO INITIATION OF SECLUSION: (Circle one response for each)

1) Decrease patient stimulation.	1) Yes	2) No
2) Planned staff presence in milieu.	1) Yes	2) No
3) Verbal de-escalation techniques.	1) Yes	2) No
4) Redirected patient to another activity.	1) Yes	2) No
5) Advised patient to stop present activity.	1) Yes	2) No
6) Advised patient that present behavior will not be tolerated.	1) Yes	2) No
7) Informed patient that present behavior will require seclusion.	1) Yes	2) No
8) Behavior plan/contract.	1) Yes	2) No
9) Team member collaboration.	1) Yes	2) No
10) Potential for possible seclusion was identified by staff.	1) Yes	2) No
11) Other		

PRN medications were given within 6 hours prior to the seclusion event: (Circle one response)
1) PRN medications were not ordered.
2) Patient refused medication.
3) PRN medications were not given.
4) PRN dose was held because of earlier dosing.
Circle one response for each statement:

PRN medications, other than Inapsine for agitation, were ordered.	1) Yes	2) No
PRN medication was given in seclusion due to patient agitation in the milieu.	1) Yes	2) No

POST-SECLUSION INTERVENTIONS: (circle one response)
PRN medications were given while patient was in seclusion:
1) 1 to 2 times per shift.   3) Less than 1 time per day.
2) 1 to 2 times per day.   4) No PRNs were given.

USE CLASS I-V CODES TO RESPOND TO QUESTIONS 1-4 BELOW: (Respond to each blank using the applicable class code)
  Class I -   No visible evidence of any physical injury, e.g., bruise,reddened areas.
  Class II -   A small scrape, abrasion, or bruise that heals without treatment in a few days.
  Class III -   A suspected bone injury requiring an x-ray but no evidence of fracture is seen.
             A laceration that requires suturing and medical treatment.
  Class IV -   A confirmed fracture of any bone or head injury (neurological injury).
  Class V -   Death

1) Outcome/injury to the patient while initiating seclusion. _____
2) Outcome/injury to the patient while in seclusion.   _____
3) Outcome/injury to staff while initiating seclusion   _____
4) Outcome/injury to staff while patient was in seclusion. _____

Additional Comments:_____

CHAPTER 11

Outcomes of Early Hospital Discharge of Women Undergoing Abdominal Hysterectomy

Andrea O. Hollingsworth

Susan M. Cohen

EDITORS' NOTE: Because of the reduction of hospital stays in recent years, many professionals predicted high readmission rates for those patients who could not recover unassisted at home. Andrea Hollingsworth at Villanova University and Susan Cohen at Yale University studied the replacement of hospital time with transitional care, using nurse practitioners to guide the home recovery of women who had undergone abdominal hysterectomy. Costs were decreased, patient satisfaction was increased, and readmission rates remained unchanged. Readers may be interested in testing this early discharge model with their own patient populations.

IDENTIFYING THE PATIENT OUTCOME

Hysterectomy is one of the most frequently performed surgical procedures among women in the United States, with 556,000 procedures performed annu-

AUTHORS' NOTE: This study was supported by Grant 1-PO1-NR01859 from the National Center for Nursing Research, National Institutes of Health.

155

ally (Bureau of the Census, 1997). This study tested a model of early hospital discharge and transitional home follow-up care in women hospitalized for abdominal hysterectomy. The model replaced a portion of hospital care with transitional home follow-up care by master's-prepared nurse practitioners. The researchers wanted to determine if this model could decrease the cost of caring for women undergoing abdominal hysterectomy while maintaining high-quality physical and psychosocial outcomes.

The selection of appropriate outcome measurements was essential to determine if the intervention of transitional care could produce the same physical and psychosocial results as those of routine hospital care. The physical outcomes were morbidity and return to normal activities. Advances in health care have improved morbidity statistics for patients undergoing hysterectomy for non-oncologic reasons. Despite these advances, women who undergo hysterectomy surgery are still at risk for complications, including infection, thromboembolic disease, hemorrhage, urinary tract infection, bladder injuries, and wound dehiscence (Harris, 1997). Selecting morbidity outcome variables proved difficult because of limitations inherent in the measurement of physical symptoms such as fever or interventions such as the administration of antibiotics. The research team decided to use unscheduled acute care visits to the surgeon or clinic and rehospitalizations as a way of comparing morbidity outcomes for each group. Extra acute care visits and rehospitalizations were a concrete measure of serious, physical complications.

The psychosocial outcomes were anxiety, depression, hostility, self-esteem, satisfaction with care, and sexual functioning. Research from the 1940s through the 1960s in the area of posthysterectomy depression confirmed the notion that women were more depressed after hysterectomy than after other kinds of surgery (Drellich & Bieber, 1958; Lindemann, 1941; Melody, 1962). Most of the recent research, however, fails to support earlier findings regarding the incidence of depression posthysterectomy. Webb and Wilson-Barnett (1983) found that depression levels were reduced after the operation, and the majority of women were glad to have had the operation. Obviously, some of the difference in the findings of posthysterectomy depression may be attributable to the time periods in which the studies were done. Societal perceptions of women and women's self-perception have evolved from the 1940s to the present.

BUILDING THE TEAM

The study was designed to discharge one group of posthysterectomy patients earlier than the routine during the time period in which the study was conducted and to provide home follow-up by a women's health practitioner. The study was a randomized clinical trial conducted during a 3-year period. The team consisted of four investigators: two principal investigators (school of nursing faculty members in the health care of women division), and two coinvestigators (a physician and a nurse practitioner from the physician's practice). The nursing intervention was provided by a full-time master's-prepared nurse practitioner and a part-time individual with the same credentials. Throughout the study, there were also two research assistants who collected the data. These were graduate students in the school of nursing in which the research was conducted.

The study was conducted as part of a program grant in which there were two other studies being carried out using the same model of care for two other patient groups. The investigators for the overall program included an economist, who analyzed the cost data outcomes.

SELECTING AN INSTRUMENT

The instruments used in this study were selected because the investigators had used them previously in similar studies or because they had been recommended by colleagues (Table 11.1). Return to normal activities was measured by the Enforced Social Dependency Scale. Enforced social dependency was defined as a state in which patients require help or assistance from other people for performing tasks that in ordinary circumstances they could perform by themselves (Fink, 1985). The original scale, developed in 1978, has been revised and tested with a variety of patient groups (Benoliel, McCorkle, & Young, 1980). Fink (1985) reported the internal consistency reliability to be 0.92 and the correlation with the Sickness Impact Profile to be 0.89. Two particular factors are measured: personal and social competence. Personal competence includes the activities of eating, dressing, walking, traveling, bathing, and toileting. Each activity is coded on a 6-point scale ranging from requiring no assistance to being completely dependent. Scores are summed, resulting in a range of 6 to 36. Social competence includes measures of activities in three areas: home, work, and social or recreational. They are rated on a 4-point scale from usual activity to no activity. Competency in communication is also included and rated on a 3-point scale. Scores are summed, resulting in a range of 4 to 15. The total score for the entire scale ranges from 10 to 51, with the higher scores reflecting greater enforced dependency.

There are several advantages to using this scale. It takes 10 to 20 minutes to administer. It is a semistructured interview guide, allowing the subject to share her perception of current activities. Also, because the first question is general and open-ended, the subject often gives enough information to allow rating on the item without resorting to additional questions. Responses are scored in a standardized way that enables comparison across time and across groups. The scale has been shown to be sensitive to change over time.

The Multiple Affect Adjective Check List–State Form, Revised (MAACL-R) was used to measure anxiety, depression, and hostility. The MAACL-R consists

TABLE 11.1 Instruments Used

Instrument	Measures	Range Possible	Validity and Reliability
Enforced Social Dependency Scale	Return to normal activity	6-36: Higher score indicates greater dependence.	Benoliel et al. (1980), Fink (1985)
Multiple Affect Adjective Checklist— State Form	Anxiety, depression, and hostility	Form contains 132 mood affect-connoting adjectives. A scoring key is provided for each area. The higher the score in each area, the greater degree of anxiety, depression, and hostility.	Lubin et al. (1986), Zuckerman et al. (1983)
Rosenberg Self-Esteem Scale	Self-esteem	10-40: Higher score indicates degree of positive self-esteem.	Rosenberg (1972), Silber and Tippett (1965)
LaMonica-Oberst Patient Satisfaction Scale	Satisfaction with care	41-205: Higher score indicates greater satisfaction with nursing care.	LaMonica et al. (1986)
Derogatis Sexual Functioning Inventory	Sexual functioning	This is a multi-dimensional measure for 10 different areas.	Derogatis and Melisaratos (1979)

of 132 affect-connoting adjectives and provides measures of self-reported moods (Zuckerman & Lubin, 1985). On the basis of additional factor analyses, the original anxiety, depression, and hostility scales were changed from bipolar scales to briefer unipolar scales. A new composite score (anxiety + depression + hostility) is labeled dysphoria. Norms for the state form of the MAACL-R have been reported for college samples by Zuckerman, Lubin, and Rinck (1983). The internal consistency estimates (coefficient alphas) are adequately high. Across the scales relevant to this study, the median internal reliability over eight samples was reported as 0.85, with a range from 0.69 to 0.95 (Lubin et al., 1986).

Self-esteem was measured with the Rosenberg Self-Esteem Scale (Rosenberg, 1972). The scale was devised to achieve a unidimensional measure of global self-regard. The scale consists of 10 items on a 4-point Likert response scale ranging from strongly agree to strongly disagree. Positively and negatively worded items are used to reduce response set. The total score reflects the degree of positive self-esteem. Silber and Tippett (1965) obtained a 2-week test-retest reliability of 0.85 for this scale and established its concurrent validity through correlation with three other measures of self-esteem. This scale was selected for use in this study because it directly measures a person's general sense of self-worth and self-acceptance and because of its ease of administration. It required 2 or 3 minutes to complete and simply required a check mark for each answer.

Satisfaction with care was measured by the LaMonica-Oberst Patient Satisfaction Scale (LaMonica, Oberst, Madea, & Wolf, 1986). This scale is a revision of the Risser scale (Risser, 1975). Although it was intended to be more reflective of care in an acute care setting, only one item (answering call lights) is limited to use in a hospital setting. The Risser scale was originally developed for use in an ambulatory care setting. Satisfaction with nursing care is defined here as "the degree of congruence between patients' expectations of nursing care and their perceptions of care actually received" (LaMonica et al., 1986, p. 43).

This tool was selected for use in the study because of the relevance of the items to the subjects in the study, the psychometric properties of the scale, and the ease with which it can be administered. The instrument contains 41 items that are rated on a 5-point scale from strongly agree to strongly disagree and can be administered in 10 to 15 minutes. The potential range of scores for the total scale is 41 to 205.

Sexual functioning was measured by the Derogatis Sexual Functioning Inventory (DSFI). The scale is a multidimensional measure for estimating the frequency, quality, and attitudes toward sexual behavior. It consists of 10 areas: information, experience, drive, attitudes, psychological symptoms, effects, gender role definition, fantasy, body image, and satisfaction (Derogatis & Melisaratos, 1979).

Reliability for the DSFI showed both internal consistency and high test-retest coefficients. The DSFI has been validated on multiple populations, including healthy and dysfunctional groups. The DSFI has been normed on male and female subjects as well as on heterosexual and homosexual subjects.

For the purpose of this study, several subscales were not used because they duplicated data from the MAACL-R and the Rosenberg Self-Esteem Scale. The subscales that were used included experience, drive, gender role definition, fantasy, body image, and satisfaction.

MEASURING THE PATIENT OUTCOMES

Research Design

Women undergoing abdominal hysterectomy for nononcologic indications in the University Medical Center associated with the school of nursing were approached to participate in the study. Following informed consent, subjects were randomly assigned to one of two groups using the sealed-envelope technique. Consent was obtained either prior to surgery or within the first 24 hours after surgery, and the physician was blinded to each patient's group assignment. Subjects were at least 21 years old, English speaking, lived within a 50-mile radius of the hospital, and had a working telephone in the home.

Women in the control group received standard postoperative care in the hospital and routine hospital discharge at a time determined by the operating surgeon. No follow-up services beyond standard postoperative office visits were provided for this group.

In the experimental group, the nurse practitioners encouraged the physicians to discharge patients early provided they met a standard set of discharge criteria, which included patient readiness for discharge and an environment supportive of convalescence at home. The protocol for early discharge included routine discharge criteria (in some cases, wound staples were still in place for removal at home by the nurse practitioner) and the absence of physiologic complications; the ability to assume self-care or to have a support person in the home able and willing to assist in care; and patient's demonstrated knowledge of reportable signs and symptoms, temperature taking, activity limitations, dietary needs, wound care, pain management, resumption of sexual activity, normal bowel function, and expected amount and duration of vaginal bleeding. The patient also demonstrated no overt emotional problems. The environment at home had to be supportive of convalescence with sufficient basic services, such as heat, telephone or ready access to one, assistance or an environment that provided opportunity for rest, and available transportation.

The nurse practitioner coordinated discharge planning with the patient, physician, hospital nursing staff, and, if appropriate, social service staff. The nurse practitioner also provided or coordinated patient teaching, helped establish a time frame for the day of discharge, coordinated plans for medical follow-up, and made referrals to community agencies when needed. When problems were encountered, the nurse consulted with the physician, social service staff, and community resource groups to resolve the situation.

Following the early discharge of patients in the experimental group, the nurse made a minimum of two home visits—the first on the day after discharge and the second within 1 week—and 10 telephone calls during 8 weeks. The purpose of the home visits and telephone contacts was to assess and monitor the physical, emotional, and functional status of the patient; provide direct care when needed; assist in obtaining services or other resources available in the community; and provide teaching, counseling, and support during the convalescent period. If complications occurred, the nurse consulted with the physician backup for a plan of immediate treatment and added additional home visits and telephone calls as necessary.

The nurse was available to patients and families by telephone from 8 a.m. to 10 p.m. Monday through Friday and from 8 a.m. to noon on Saturday and Sunday, and the nurse had backup from physicians familiar with the patient. After 10 p.m. on weekdays and after noon on weekends, patients were asked to call their private physicians or the hospital emergency room should there be a need for immediate care.

Comparison of outcomes and cost of health care was made between the control and experimental groups during the postoperative period. Physical outcomes were determined by keeping track of any additional acute care visits and rehospitalizations that patients experienced. An acute care visit was defined as a visit to the physician's office, clinic, or emergency room outside of the routine postoperative care. In addition, return to normal activities was measured. Psychosocial outcomes that were measured included anxiety, depression, hostility, self-esteem, sexual functioning, and satisfaction with care.

Research assistants collected the data beginning when the subject was still in the hospital. Arrangements were then made for the research assistant to contact the subject by phone to do the remainder of the data collection. All other data were gathered through phone calls. The research tools were chosen with this in mind. Measures of anxiety, depression, hostility, and self-esteem were done during hospitalization and at 1, 4, and 8 weeks postdischarge. Return to normal activities information was collected at 2, 4, and 8 weeks postdischarge. Data on sexual functioning were gathered at postoperative weeks 4 and 8. Satisfaction with nursing care was measured once at 8 weeks after discharge. All research assistants received training in using these various research tools, particularly the Enforced Social Dependency Scale. This required the assistant to interpret the subjects' answers and place them on a scale of activities.

Information concerning morbidity, acute care visits, and rehospitalizations was gathered from chart review and patient interviews.

The administration of these measurement tools did not present any difficulties. There was a problem in contacting the subjects while they recuperated because they tended to be out of their homes more often and it took 45 minute to 1 hour to collect all the information. In general, the research assistants found the tools easy to use, and subjects had little difficulty answering the questions.

TABLE 11.2 Benign Indications for Hysterectomy

Diagnosis	Early Discharge (n = 54)	Control (n = 59)
Myomas	32	35
Cervical intraepithelial neoplasia	4	3
Dysfunctional uterine bleeding	3	4
Endometriosis	1	4
Prolapse	1	0
Severe pelvic inflammatory disease	0	1
Endometrial cancer Stage I	1	0
Other	12	12

ANALYZING THE DATA

Frequency distributions and summary statistics were calculated for all study variables. Evidence of initial equivalence of experimental and control groups was assessed on the demographic variables by unpaired *t* tests or chi-square. Chi-square was used to compare the two groups when the dependent variable was categorical, as in rehospitalizations. When the dependent variable was continuous, and measured more than once, analysis of variance (ANOVA) with repeated measures was used. These variables included the number of acute care visits, return to normal activities, anxiety, depression, hostility, self-esteem, and sexual functioning. The researchers attempted to determine whether the two groups differed on these variables and what changes occurred over time.

SUMMARIZING THE FINDINGS

The sample included 113 women who underwent an abdominal hysterectomy—54 in the early discharge group and 59 in the control group. Table 11.2 displays the number of women in the study and the indications for surgery. There were no statistically significant differences between the groups in terms of age, educational level, marital status, race, hospital insurance, annual income, or occupational level (Table 11.3).

Physical Outcomes

There were no statistically significant differences between the groups in terms of postoperative acute care visits, rehospitalizations, or infections

TABLE 11.3 Demographic Data

Characteristic	Early Discharge (n = 54)	Control (n = 59)
Mean age ± SD	47.6 ± 10.5	47.5 ± 9.9
Educational level		
High school or less	38%	30%
Part college or college graduate	44%	46%
Graduate degree	15%	25%
Marital status		
Never married	15%	17%
Married	61%	61%
Divorced/separated/widowed	24%	22%
Race		
White	64%	67%
African American	36%	33%
Hospital insurance		
Private	90%	88%
Public	10%	12%
Income		
$17,000-$24,500	22%	19%
$25,000-$34,500	19%	14%
$35,000-$50,000	16%	21%
$50,000-$75,000	19%	17%
More than $75,000	24%	29%
Occupational level		
Skilled	61%	55%
Minor professional/professional	39%	45%

($\chi^2 = 3.57$, $df = 1$, $.05 < p < .10$). The early discharge group, however, demonstrated a trend for fewer postoperative acute care visits. In the early discharge group, 3 subjects had 7 acute care visits, whereas in the control group 10 subjects had 19 visits.

On measures of return to normal activities, there were no significant differences between groups when compared using repeated measures ANOVA. Personal and social dependency scores for both groups demonstrated a similar trend over time. These scores were highest in the immediate postoperative period and then decreased over time. Personal dependency scores and social dependency scores were highest at 2 weeks postsurgery and then decreased significantly between 2 weeks and 4 weeks postoperatively ($p < .001$) and decreased again between 4 and 8 weeks postoperatively ($p < .001$).

Psychosocial Outcomes

There were no statistically significant differences between the early discharge group and the control group in measures of anxiety, depression, and self-esteem. Anxiety, depression, and hostility were highest in the immediate postoperative period and decreased over the period of 8 weeks. The scores for both anxiety and depression decreased significantly between hospitalization and 1 week postsurgery, between 1 week and 4 weeks postsurgery, and between 4 weeks and 8 weeks (all significant at $p < .001$). Hostility also decreased significantly between hospitalization and 1 week postsurgery ($t = 2.26$, $p < .05$), but hostility scores did not change significantly at the remaining data points. Data obtained from the Rosenberg Self-Esteem Scale were limited due to lack of variability.

There was a significant difference between the early discharge group and the control group in satisfaction with care, with the women in the early discharge group being more satisfied with their nursing care (Figure 11.1)

Cost Outcomes

The experimental group was discharged a mean of one half day earlier than the control group at a savings of 6% of total cost. The cost included the expense of the nurse practitioner's time in the early discharge group. The nurse practitioner's time was calculated on an hourly basis that included the time used in giving care, traveling, completing documentation, and counseling by phone.

To compare differences in cost, the research team, particularly the economist, used hospital charges. The informed consent contained permission for the hospital to release a copy of the charges to the investigators.

APPLYING THE FINDINGS TO PRACTICE

In today's health care environment, with ever shorter hospital stays, it is important to determine a program of care that can ensure similar outcomes to those

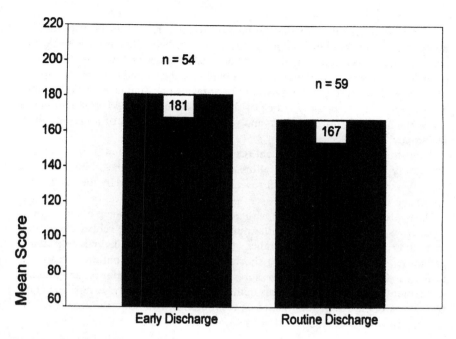

Figure 11.1. Satisfaction With Care (Range Possible, 41-205; Higher Score Indicates Greater Satisfaction [$(t = 3.03, p < .01)$])

of the traditional hospital stays of only a few years ago. A program of early hospital discharge and transitional care for women who have undergone abdominal hysterectomy has the potential to decrease iatrogenic illness and hospital-acquired infection, increase a woman's satisfaction with her health care, and decrease hospital and postoperative costs. With the continuing emphasis on providing cost-conscious but comprehensive health and illness care, such programs are an economic necessity.

On the basis of the findings, the researchers concluded that early hospital discharge of postoperative hysterectomy patients, according to the model used in this study, is safe, feasible, and cost-effective. In addition, it provided continuity of care. Women in the early discharge group were significantly more satisfied with their care than the women in the control group. This hospital-based approach has several advantages: It provides continuity of care by using a master's-prepared nurse, who has a specialized knowledge of women's health care; it includes the nurse as an integral part of the hospital staff who is familiar with the protocols and teaching plan used by the hospital; and it allows the patient and her family access to the nurse 7 days a week.

The researchers believe that home follow-up care should be provided by nurses who have specialized knowledge of women's health care because of the specific needs of these women. This knowledge is necessary to make the appropriate assessments and interventions in physical care and to intervene appropriately with teaching and counseling in areas of emotional and psychosocial adjustments. Hysterectomy is one of the most commonly performed surgeries for women in the United States, and there is no indication of a decline in its frequency.

The study also supported recent research that indicates that, following hysterectomy, women experience feelings of well-being rather than depression and anxiety as was believed in earlier research. This is supported by the research of Lambden et al. (1997).

The safety of early discharge with transitional care follow-up by nurse practitioners is supported by the similar number of postoperative rehospitalizations in each group and the fewer number of acute care visits in the early discharge group. As the concern regarding shorter hospital stays and patient dissatisfaction with their care continues to increase, it may be beneficial for hospitals to implement models of care such as demonstrated in this study. A hospital could provide safe, improved, extended care to women and their families as they experience this very common but serious surgery.

PLANNING FUTURE PATIENT OUTCOMES PROJECTS

In the environment of today's changing health care system, the average length of hospital stay following abdominal hysterectomy has been decreasing nationally. Unfortunately, there is a dearth of literature concerning the outcomes of women sent home with little preparation or follow-up after this surgery. This type of study on the outcomes of early discharge following abdominal hysterectomy is increasingly important as we strive to deliver quality care in a cost-effective manner. Further study is required to more fully understand the effects of early discharge following hysterectomy on women and their families.

REFERENCES

Benoliel, J., McCorkle, R., & Young, K. (1980). Development of a social dependency scale. *Research in Nursing and Health, 3,* 3-10.

Bureau of the Census. (1997). *Statistical abstract of the United States* (117th ed.). Washington, DC: U.S. Department of Commerce.

Derogatis, L., & Melisaratos, N. (1979). The DSFI: A multidimensional measure of sexual functioning. *Journal of Marital Therapy, 5,* 244-281.

Drellich, M., & Bieber, I. (1958). Psychologic importance of the uterus. *Journal of Nervous and Mental Disorders, 126,* 322-336.

Fink, A. (1985). *Social dependency and self-care agency: A descriptive-correlational study of ALS patients.* Unpublished thesis, University of Washington, Seattle.

Harris, W. J. (1997). Complications of hysterectomy. *Clinical Obstetrics and Gynecology, 40*(4), 928-938.

Lambden, M. P., Bellamy, G., Ogburn-Russell, L., Preece, C. K., Moore, S., Pepin, T., Croop, J., & Culbert, G. (1997). Women's sense of well-being before and after hysterectomy. *Journal of Obstetrical, Gynecological, and Neonatal Nursing, 26*(5), 540-548.

LaMonica, E., Oberst, M., Madea, A., & Wolf, R. (1986). Development of a patient satisfaction scale. *Research in Nursing and Health, 9,* 43-50.

Lindemann, E. (1941). Observations of psychiatric sequelae to surgical operations in women. *American Journal of Psychiatry, 98,* 132.

Lubin, B., Zuckerman, M., Hanson, P., Armstrong, T., Rinch, C., & Seever, M. (1986). Reliability and validity of the Multiple Affect Adjective Check List-Revised. *Journal of Psychopathology and Behavioral Assessment, 8*(2), 103-128.

Melody, G. (1962). Depressive reactions following hysterectomy. *American Journal of Obstetrics and Gynecology, 83,* 413.

Risser, N. (1975). Development of an instrument to measure patient satisfaction with nurses and nursing care in primary care settings. *Nursing Research, 24,* 45-52.

Rosenberg, M. (1972). *Society and the adolescent self-image.* Princeton, NJ: Princeton University Press.

Silber, E., & Tippett, J. (1965). Self-esteem: Clinical assessment and measurement validation. *Psychological Reports, 16,* 1017-1071.

Webb, C., & Wilson-Barnett, J. (1983). Self concept, social support and hysterectomy. *International Journal of Nursing Studies, 20,* 97.

Zuckerman, M., & Lubin, B. (1985). *Manual for the Multiple Affect Adjective Check List* (Rev. ed.). San Diego: Educational and Industrial Testing Service.

Zuckerman, M., Lubin, B., & Rinck, C. (1983). Construction of new scales for the Multiple Affect Adjective Check List. *Journal of Behavioral Assessment, 5,* 119-129.

CHAPTER 12

Swimming and Central Venous Catheter-Related Infections in Children With Cancer

Jacqueline Robbins

Philene Cromwell

David N. Korones

EDITORS' NOTE: This chapter will help the reader seeking to measure patient outcomes in many ways. First, the writers challenge readers to use outcomes data not traditionally used to guide patient care. Second, they demonstrate ethical conflicts that can occur when examining patient outcomes. Randomly assigning children with central venous catheters to a swim or nonswim group to determine which group would have more infections was clearly not in the best interest of the children. Instead, this multidisciplinary team chose a retrospective study with parental reports of swimming behaviors with central venous catheters in the past. Finally, the authors take the reader through the steps they went through in deciding how to analyze these patient data. Should children who swam only once be included with the group of nonswimmers or the group of frequent swimmers? Anyone who must measure a difficult patient outcome will benefit from this chapter.

IDENTIFYING THE PATIENT OUTCOME

Perhaps the greatest advance in the supportive care of children undergoing treatment for cancer is the indwelling central venous catheter. This catheter is essential for the administration of chemotherapy, infusion of intravenous fluids and other medications, and withdrawal of blood samples. Although the catheter is an integral part of care in pediatric oncology and significantly adds to the quality of life of the child with cancer, it is not without its risks. These risks include the formation of a clot at the tip of the catheter, malfunctioning or breaking of the catheter, and development of infections around or within the catheter (Tobiansky et al., 1997). Infection is probably the most frequently encountered complication. Infections can be caused by bacteria entering the catheter tunnel from the exit site (the point at which the catheter exits from under the skin) or bacteria entering the catheter lumen at the access site (the point through which blood is drawn and fluids are infused) (Raad & Bodey, 1992).

Although there have been many studies of the potential risk factors for catheter-related infections, none have specifically examined swimming as one of these factors (Kellerman et al., 1996; Press, Ramsey, Larson, Fefer, & Hickman, 1984). Despite the lack of data, clinicians are concerned that swimming may increase the risk of catheter-related infections. Therefore, many oncologists advise that children with indwelling catheters refrain from swimming. Because there are no data to substantiate this concern and because swimming is such an important activity for these children, we decided to survey families of children with cancer to determine whether there was indeed an association between swimming and catheter-related infection.

Although at the time of this study our institution maintained a "no-swim policy" for children with cancer and indwelling catheters, many children did swim. In working with these children and families, it was evident that allowing the children to swim would enhance their quality of life. This became particularly clear when we spent time at a summer camp for children with cancer. The camp is located on a lake and has its own swimming pool. Some of the camp's most popular activities for the children are the pool parties and beachfront activities. It was difficult for us to restrict the children with catheters from these activities when we had no data on which to base this restriction. Spending time with these children outside of the hospital setting and seeing firsthand how this restriction affected them provided the impetus for us to reevaluate our policy. Maximizing the quality of life of the children we care for is always a priority. Hence, we decided that we needed to provide data to either support our current policies or to make changes in our recommendations.

BUILDING THE TEAM

Our team for this project consisted of three members of the division of pediatric hematology/oncology—two advanced practice nurses and one attending physician. After spending a week as the nurse at the previously mentioned camp, one of the advanced practice nurses became particularly interested in conducting research to determine whether swimming did indeed put children with catheters at increased risk of infection. She then invited me, a pediatric nurse practitioner, to join her in the clinical research project.

Because both of us were novices at clinical research, we asked one of our attending physicians with an extensive background in clinical research to assist us with the process, particularly the methodology and data analysis. The attending physician was also very interested in answering this question and agreed to join our research team. The three of us had several meetings to refine the study questions and to determine the best study design. We decided that the best way to obtain the necessary information would be a self-report questionnaire for patients and families. We decided to target patients who had catheters in place within the 2 years prior to this study. This time frame would produce a sufficient number of participants to conduct the study without having to go back so far in time that patients and families would not be able to remember information accurately. We also discussed the division of responsibilities for implementing the study and created a time line for completing specific steps of the research process. The responsibilities were divided as discussed in the following sections.

Advanced Practice Nurses

Our first responsibility was to develop a proposal, including the questionnaire created for this study, to be submitted to the institutional review board (IRB) at our institution. In preparing this proposal, we developed an information sheet for patients and families to support informed consent. Following IRB approval, we distributed and collected questionnaires, collected data from the medical record, entered data, and composed the written research report (Robbins, Cromwell, & Korones, 1999).

Attending Physician

The attending physician functioned as a mentor to the two advanced practice nurses throughout the entire process and was specifically responsible for developing the methodology and conducting the statistical analyses after the data were collected.

SELECTING AN INSTRUMENT

We decided to measure outcomes using a self-administered questionnaire that we developed specifically for this project (see Appendix A). Before designing this questionnaire, we identified the information necessary to answer our research question. We believed that it would be important to obtain as much information as possible about the child's swimming habits—that is, not only whether they swam but also how often, where, when, and how they cared for their catheters after swimming. We also decided that it was equally important to explore other potential and confounding risk factors for infection, such as age, diagnosis, general catheter care, bathing habits, and catheter care at the time of bathing.

With these factors in mind, we designed a questionnaire that covered four broad areas: (a) demographic data and clinical variables, such as gender, age, diagnosis, catheter type, date the catheter was inserted and removed, and number of catheters placed during treatment; (b) swimming habits and catheter care before and after swimming; (c) bathing habits and catheter care at the time of bathing; and (d) general daily catheter care (e.g., frequency of catheter flushing, catheter dressing changes, and type of dressing used).

As we developed the questionnaire and information sheet, we faced the dilemma of whether patients and families should be aware of our central hypothesis. We were concerned that if they knew we were searching for a correlation between swimming and infection, it might influence how they answered the questions. We considered keeping the participants blind to the purpose of this study and dispersing questions about swimming among other unrelated questions within the questionnaire. We believed, however, that our families would very quickly figure out the central hypothesis of this study; they are sophisticated in their knowledge of medical issues, and swimming in particular has been a long-standing issue of contention and a topic of much discussion. Furthermore, because we have a very close relationship with most of the families, and several of them had already admitted to swimming, we believed they would be honest in their answers. For these reasons, we decided to inform patients and families of the true purpose of the study.

There were a few weaknesses inherent in the survey approach that potentially could have affected the accuracy of the answers in our study. One consideration was the retrospective design of the self-report questionnaire. Patients and families were being asked to recall information from 1 to 2 years prior to completing the questionnaire. Their inability to remember correctly may have affected the accuracy of their responses. Another concern was whether families would answer honestly; because we have a no-swim policy, patients and their families may not have felt comfortable confessing that they had violated this policy. As previously mentioned, however, we were confident that most of them would answer truthfully.

Another difficulty with our questionnaire was that, due to its retrospective design, we were unable to establish exact dates of when children went swimming. We were only able to determine the seasons during which the children swam. Therefore, although we were able to determine whether a child went swimming and developed an infection within the same season, we were unable to determine precisely whether the infection occurred before or after swimming.

A final issue was the need to modify the questionnaire. After we reviewed the first 10 questionnaires and talked to the parent respondents, we learned that some questions were confusing, others had inappropriate multiple-choice answers, and a few questions needed to be added. We learned from this the importance of piloting a questionnaire on a small group of subjects before distributing it to the entire study population.

MEASURING THE PATIENT OUTCOME

Catheter Infection

The major outcome examined in this study was catheter-related infections. Because there are different types of catheter infections, and because there can be subjectivity in diagnosing such infections, it was imperative for us to define the main types of catheter infections at the outset: (a) exit site, (b) tunnel, and (c) intraluminal infections. We obtained established definitions from previous studies and used these definitions to determine whether our patients had catheter infections.

Swimming as a Risk Factor

We were interested in whether swimming in general was associated with an increase in catheter-related infections or whether only certain aspects of swimming increased the risk of infection. To determine this, we first asked if the child ever swam with his or her catheter in place. If the answer to this question was yes, we asked about the type of water in which the child swam, the season(s) during which he or she swam, the type of precautions taken to care for the catheter before and after swimming, and the frequency of swimming. We wondered if infection might be more likely to occur in children who swam frequently when compared with those who swam only once.

Other Risk Factors

It was just as important to measure accurately any other postulated risk factors for infection. We knew that there might be other factors associated with catheter infections that might confound our ability to interpret any association between swimming and catheter-related infections. We therefore included demographics in the questionnaire. For example, we obtained demographic data such as gender and age to determine whether certain groups of children were more likely to engage in swimming activities based on these characteristics. We also examined specific diagnoses to determine whether diagnosis played a role in the child's risk of developing an infection. We further inquired about general daily catheter care (dressing changes, hub changes, flushing, and the person caring for the catheter) to determine whether differences in this care had any impact on the incidence of catheter-related infections. Finally, we included questions regarding bathing habits and catheter care around the time of bathing to help us determine whether different approaches to bathing affected the incidence of catheter-related infections in these children. For example, do children who submerge their catheters in bathwater have a higher incidence of infection than those who are sponge-bathed?

The questionnaire was distributed to families during their visits to the outpatient pediatric oncology clinic or mailed to their homes. Families were provided with an information sheet explaining the purpose of this study. This sheet also stated that their participation was voluntary, that they could withdraw at any time, that no judgment or criticism would be directed toward them if they admitted to swimming, and that all responses would be kept confidential.

One potential barrier in conducting this study was having too few families return the questionnaire. Low response rates of self-administered questionnaires can pose methodological problems—for example, are there inherent differences between responders and nonresponders such that the responders are not truly representative of the group being studied? The best way to circumvent this problem is to get everyone to respond. Our two advanced practice nurses followed up with telephone calls to the families who had not returned their questionnaires. This ultimately resulted in a greater than 90% response rate. We attributed our success to the close personal relationships we had with the families.

Once all the questionnaires were returned, each response to a question was numerically coded. When the coding was completed, the results were entered into a Microsoft Excel spreadsheet (1997). Basic calculations, such as means and medians, were performed using this program. Other analyses were performed on the Graph Pad Instat statistical package (1998).

ANALYZING THE DATA

Our analysis focused on differences between the children who swam and those who did not. The results of this analysis are summarized in Table 12.1. We first examined and compared basic demographic data: the number of children and number of catheters among the swimmers and nonswimmers, the median age

TABLE 12.1 Differences Between Swimmers and Nonswimmers

	Swimmers	*Nonswimmers*	*Significance*[a]
Number of children	49	46	
Number of catheters	50	51	
Age (years), median	9	8	*ns*[1]
Months catheter in place, median	14	7	*p* = .001[1]
Total infections/catheter	34/50 (.68)	13/51 (.26)	*p* < .001[2]
Tunnel or exit infections/catheter	14/50 (.28)	8/51 (.16)	*ns*[2]
Bloodstream infections/catheter	20/50 (.40)	5/51 (.10)	*p* = .001[2]
Total infections/month	34/843 (.04)	13/506 (.025)	RR = 1.6[3] (*ns*)
Tunnel or exit infections/month	20/843 (.02)	8/506 (.016)	RR = 1.5[3] (*ns*)
Bloodstream infections/month	14/843 (.016)	5/506 (.009)	RR = 1.7[3] (*ns*)
Summer months catheter in place, median	4	2	*p* = .001[1]
Summer infections/summer month	15/220 (.06)	6/123 (.05)	RR = 1.4[3] (*ns*)
Summer tunnel or exit infections/ summer month	7/220 (.03)	4/123 (.03)	RR = 1.0[3] (*ns*)
Summer bloodstream infections/ summer month	8/220 (.03)	2/123 (.016)	RR = 2.2[3] (*ns*)

a. *ns,* Not significant; RR, risk ratio; 1, Mann-Whitney *U* test; 2, chi-square test; 3, significance based on 95% confidence interval (see text).

of the children in each group, and the median number of months catheters were in place for children in each group.

We then focused on the main issue—rates of catheter-related infections in swimmers compared to nonswimmers. We first examined the crude rate of such infections as measured by total number of infections per total number of catheters. We used the chi-square test for this comparison. With this crude analysis, we found a higher rate of infections in the swimmers than in the nonswimmers (Table 12.1). When we further examined the specific types of catheter infec-

tions of these children, we found that crude rates of bloodstream catheter infections were higher among the swimmers; the rates of exit site or tunnel infections, however, were the same in the two groups.

Simply examining crude rates of infection did not tell the whole story. Such
rates needed to be adjusted for other factors that may have affected the rates
(Fleiss, 1981). For example, we noticed that, on average, the swimmers had
their catheters in place twice as long as the nonswimmers (Table 12.1). Thus,
the swimmers may have had a higher rate of infection simply because they had
their catheters in longer and not because they went swimming. To adjust for this
possibility, we measured rates of infection as infections per catheter-month
(i.e., the total number of infections per total number of months children had
their catheters in place). We then compared rates between swimmers and
nonswimmers with a standard test of comparison of rates, the risk ratio (relative
risk). The risk ratio is a comparison of risks between two groups. For example,
in Table 12.1, when we compare the risk of infections per month in the swimmers (0.04) to the nonswimmers (0.025), the risk ratio is 0.04 to 0.025 or 1.5.
Thus, there is a 1.5-fold increased risk of infection in swimmers versus nonswimmers. To determine whether this increase was statistically significant, we
calculated the 95% confidence interval; for this particular ratio, the interval is
0.8 to 2.8. This means that there is a 95% chance that the risk of infection in
swimmers versus nonswimmers is between 0.8 and 2.8. Whenever this confidence interval includes 1.0 (i.e., no difference in risk between the two groups),
the risk is considered not statistically significant. Thus, there is not a statistically
significant difference in rates of infection per month between swimmers and
nonswimmers.

We still needed to adjust for the time of year during which the infection
occurred. In our questionnaire, we had asked our patients what time of year they
went swimming; all of them swam in the summer. Thus, it seemed that if swimming were truly associated with infections, the infections would occur at
approximately the time the children went swimming (i.e., in the summer). It
made no sense that an infection in January would be associated with swimming
in July. Hence, we made a second adjustment and considered only summertime
infections.

Finally, we needed to make one more adjustment. Because we were examining only summertime infections, we needed to count only summer months for
the time children had catheters in place. When we compared the median number of summer months during which children had catheters in place, we again
found that swimmers had their catheters in place during twice as many summer
months as did the nonswimmers (Table 12.1).

With all these adjustments, we were able to obtain data on summertime infections during summer months. This enabled us to assess rates of catheter

TABLE 12.2 Differences Between Frequent Swimmers and Infrequent or
Nonswimmers

	Frequent Swimmers	*Infrequent or Nonswimmers*	*Significance*[a]
Number of children	35	60	
Number of catheters	35	66	
Age (years), median	9	8	ns^1
Months, catheter in place, median	15.5	9	$p = .038^1$
Total infections/catheter	19/35 (.54)	27/66 (.41)	ns^2
Tunnel or exit infections/catheter	6/35 (.17)	16/66 (.24)	ns^2
Bloodstream infections/catheter	13/35 (.37)	11/66 (.17)	$p = .04^2$
Total infections/month	19/579 (.03)	27/770 (.03)	$RR = 0.9^3$ (*ns*)
Tunnel or exit infections/month	6/579 (.01)	16/770 (.02)	$RR = 0.5^3$ (*ns*)
Bloodstream infections/month	13/579 (.02)	11/770 (.014)	$RR = 1.6^3$ (*ns*)
Summer months catheter in place, median	3	3	ns^1
Summer infections/summer months	8/149 (.05)	13/194 (.06)	$RR = 0.81^3$ (*ns*)
Summer tunnel or exit infections/ summer month	2/149 (.01)	9/194 (.04)	$RR = 0.3^3$ (*ns*)
Summer bloodstream infections/ summer month	6/149 (.04)	4/194 (.02)	$RR = 1.9^3$ (*ns*)

a. *ns,* Not significant; RR, risk ratio; 1, Mann-Whitney *U* test; 2, chi-square test; 3, significance based on 95% confidence interval (see text).

infections at a time children actually went swimming and compare them to rates of infection during the same time period for children who did not go swimming. The unit of comparison was summertime catheter-related infections per summertime month in the swimmers versus the nonswimmers (Table 12.1). We again used the risk ratio. This was our "bottom-line" measure of assessing swimming as a risk factor for catheter infection. It revealed no difference in rates of infection.

We decided to examine not only swimmers versus nonswimmers in our analysis but also frequent swimmers versus infrequent swimmers plus non-swimmers. Our rationale for this latter analysis was that infrequent swimmers, arbitrarily defined as children who swam less than once a month, might be more similar to those children who did not swim at all than those who swam frequently. We performed the same analyses with the same adjustments that were discussed previously. The results of these analyses are displayed in Table 12.2 and follow the same sequence as that in Table 12.1. We again found no difference in rates of infection in swimmers versus infrequent swimmers and nonswimmers.

Finally, we realized that there are other factors that might contribute to the risk of catheter-related infections, such as age of the child, diagnosis, and catheter care. We therefore compared the groups of swimmers and nonswimmers with respect to age, diagnosis, frequency of flushes, dressing changes, hub changes, type of dressing, and frequency and type of bathing. We used the chi-square and Fisher's Exact test for proportions and the Student t test and Mann-Whitney U test for comparison of means and medians, respectively. This enabled us to determine that there were no demographic factors affecting our results.

SUMMARIZING THE FINDINGS

Study findings demonstrated that there was not a higher incidence of catheter-related infections in children who swam when compared with those who did not. Because of the limitations discussed earlier, however, we believed we needed to interpret these results with caution before changing our clinical practice.

APPLYING THE FINDINGS
TO PRACTICE

We discussed the project results at the annual retreat of the division of pediatric hematology/oncology. Those attending the retreat included the chief of the division, all the attending physicians, advanced practice nurses, laboratory researchers, and the psychosocial team. After presentation and discussion of our results, the group believed that, despite some limitations of the study, we had demonstrated no clear association between swimming and catheter-related infections. The consensus was that we had enough data to support changing our current no-swim policy.

As of the summer of 1998, children with tunneled catheters are permitted to swim. This policy has implications for the nursing staff that work with these children and families; education related to proper catheter care at the time of swimming is essential. The questionnaire for this study asked about how the child cared for his or her catheter before and after swimming. From the responses, we were able to determine that almost all the children took adequate precautions in taking care of the catheter prior to and following swimming. We believe that these precautions played a significant role in minimizing the risk of infection.

PLANNING FUTURE PATIENT OUTCOMES PROJECTS

Because the results of our research study have resulted in a change in one of our long-standing policies, it is imperative that we continue to track rates of catheter-related infections in swimmers. This will enable us to evaluate the results of our research study in everyday clinical practice. If we document an increase in rates of catheter-related infection after the children are permitted to swim, it will warrant a reassessment of our new policy and perhaps a more comprehensive prospective study of this issue.

In this study, we found that there was a higher overall incidence of catheter-related infections in children during the summer months than in other seasons, regardless of their swimming habits. This raises questions about other factors associated with the summer—for example, children perspiring more and more outdoor activity that may increase the risk of infection. Future studies should be prospective in examining these factors.

REFERENCES

Excel Version 97 Windows [Computer software]. (1997). Redmond, WA: Microsoft.

Fleiss, J. L. (1981). *Statistical methods for rates and proportions* (2nd ed.). New York: John Wiley.

Graph Pad InStat. Version 3.0 for Windows 95 [Computer software]. (1998) San Diego: Graph Pad Software.

Kellerman, S., Shay, D. K., Howard, J., Goes, C., Feusner, J., Rosenberg, J., Vugia, D. J., & Jarvis, W. R. (1996). Bloodstream infections in home infusion patients: The influence of race and needleless intravascular access devices. *Journal of Pediatrics, 129,* 711-717.

Press, O. W., Ramsey, P. G., Larson, E. B., Fefer, A., & Hickman, R. O. (1984). Hickman catheter infections in patients with malignancies. *Medicine, 63,* 189-200.

Raad, I. I., & Bodey, G. P. (1992). Infectious complications of indwelling vascular catheters. *Clinical Infectious Diseases, 15,* 197-208.

Robbins, J., Cromwell, P., & Korones, D. (1999). Swimming and central venous catheter-related infections in children with cancer. *Journal of Pediatric Oncology Nursing, 16*(1), 51-56.

Tobiansky, R., Lui, K., Dalton, D. M., Shaw, P., Martin, H., & Isaacs, D. (1997). Complications of central venous access devices in children with and without cancer. *Journal of Paediatrics & Child Health, 33,* 509-514.

CENTRAL VENOUS CATHETERS
SWIMMING: INCIDENCE OF INFECTION

Name: _____

Sex: _____ Type of catheter: _____

Age: _____ Date catheter was placed: _____

Dx: _____

Please take time to answer the following questions. Thank you.

1. Have you ever gone swimming since your Broviac catheter was put in?

   Yes ☐   No ☐

   If so, where do you swim? (check as many as are appropriate)
   Private pool ☐   Public pool ☐   Lake ☐   Pond ☐   Other ☐

2. How often do you swim?
   >1/week ☐   Once a week ☐   Once every 2 weeks ☐   Once a month ☐

3. Do you take any special precautions or special care of your catheter in preparation for swimming?   Yes ☐   No ☐

   What time of year do you usually swim? (check as many as apply)
   Summer ☐   Fall ☐   Spring ☐   Winter ☐

   If yes, please state how you care for your catheter._____

---

4. Do you take any special precautions or care of your catheter after you swim?

   Yes ☐   No ☐

   If yes, please state how you care for your catheter. _____

   _____

   _____

   If yes, how soon do you care for your catheter after you swim?

   0-1 hour ☐   1-3 hours ☐   >3 hours ☐

5. Have you ever had any redness, tenderness, and/or drainage around your
   catheter site?   Yes ☐   No ☐

   If yes, did you make any changes in how you normally care for the
   catheter site? Please state. _____

   _____

6. Were you ever placed on oral antibiotics or was antibiotic applied to the
   catheter site for local infection?   Yes ☐   No ☐

7. At any time were you admitted to the hospital for i.v. antibiotic therapy
   for an infection of your Broviac?   Yes ☐   No ☐

   If yes, when?_____

   _____

   If you have ever had any type of Broviac infection, how recently had you
   been swimming before getting the infection?

   <1 week ☐   1-2 weeks ☐   >2 weeks ☐
        Don't remember ☐   Not applicable ☐

8. Is this your first central venous catheter?   Yes ☐   No ☐
   If no, how many catheters have you previously had? _____

9. Were any of your catheters removed as a result of infection?

   Yes ☐   No ☐

10. How often do you change the dressing?

Every day ☐   Every other day ☐   Every week ☐   Every month ☐
Other ☐ _____

11. What type of dressing do you use?

Gauze ☐   Tegaderm ☐   Other ☐

12. Please describe your dressing change technique. _____

_____

_____

13. How often do you change the catheter hubs?

Every day ☐   Every other day ☐   Every week ☐   Every month ☐
Other ☐ _____

14. How often do you flush the catheter?

Every day ☐   Every other day ☐   Every week ☐   Every month ☐
Other ☐ _____

15. Who usually cares for your catheter? (check as many as are appropriate)

You ☐   Dad ☐   Mom ☐   Community health nurse ☐
Other ☐ _____

16. Which of the following bathing methods do you use? (check as many as
are appropriate)

Sponge ☐   Tub bath ☐   Shower ☐

17. How often do you bathe?

>1/week ☐   Once a week ☐   Once every 2 weeks ☐

18. Do you take any special precautions or special care of your catheter in
preparation for bathing?   Yes ☐   No ☐

19. Do you take any special precautions or care of your catheter after you
    bathe?   Yes ❑   No ❑

    If yes, please state how you care for your catheter. _____
    _____

    If yes, how soon do you care for your catheter after you bathe?
         0-1 hour ❑   1-3 hours ❑   >3 hours ❑

CHAPTER 13

Measurement of Urinary Continence Recovery Following Radical Prostatectomy

Penny Marschke

EDITORS' NOTE: This chapter provides a good example of the importance of carefully considering how to measure the outcome of interest. Should an objective measure of incontinence or patients' perception of the incontinence be used? What is an objective measure of incontinence? Would mailed surveys or telephone interviews be the best method to collect the data? The graphic displays of the data in this chapter are also useful. A pie chart and table summarize frequency data. A bar chart depicts the frequency of incontinence over time in the postoperative period.

IDENTIFYING THE PATIENT OUTCOME

The most dreaded effect of the radical prostatectomy is urinary incontinence (Walsh & Worthington, 1995). In an effort to prevent this negative outcome, medical research has focused on the impact of the surgical procedure on urinary incontinence. Nursing research has concentrated on how patients manage urinary incontinence and the effectiveness of exercises and other behavioral strategies to help patients remain dry.

For the localized prostate cancer patient and his family, the literature contains significant discrepancies about the outcome of radical prostatectomy and its effect on urinary incontinence. Gittes (1991) noted that radical prostatectomy causes permanent urinary incontinence in 2% to 4% of patients, whereas Fowler et al. (1988) documented urinary incontinence up to 32%. These reported wide ranges in the level of urinary incontinence make it difficult for a patient and his family to gauge what the outcomes of a radical prostatectomy might be for him.

As the clinical research coordinator, I provide patient teaching in the urology outpatient clinic. Patients frequently ask how long they will remain incontinent following surgery and are dissatisfied to learn only that, in our experience, incontinence is very individualized. Patients' desire for more concrete information about incontinence was one of the motivating factors behind our decision to study incontinence following radical prostatectomy. The ultimate goal was to be able to share the results of this study with prospective patients and their families.

BUILDING THE TEAM

Although a descriptive study of incontinence was a departure from the more surgically focused studies in the urology department, there was one study that was easily expanded to include this descriptive component. One of the urologists was interested in how the patient's urethral length, bladder capacity, and bladder wall thickness affect urinary continence. Combining both studies allowed for a detailed examination of this problem.

The remainder of this chapter focuses on the process of designing an instrument for the measurement of urinary continence following radical prostatectomy. Data collection and data analysis are discussed. Also, the impact this project has had on other departmental research endeavors is reviewed.

SELECTING AN INSTRUMENT

Because radical prostatectomy is the most frequently performed surgery at our institution, obtaining an adequate sample size was not a problem. Because the majority of these patients would not be returning to our institution for follow-up care, however, communicating with them after surgery required careful planning.

Methods of Administering the Questionnaire

The urologist and I decided that we would use a questionnaire to measure incontinence (Appendix A). We planned to administer it at multiple times during the postoperative period to capture the dynamic data on regaining continence. Time, resources, patient burden, and the quality of data are the major concerns when deciding on a method of administering a questionnaire.

Although mailing is relatively inexpensive and time efficient, enormous concerns exist about the return rate of the questionnaires. Therefore, we decided that phoning each of the patients and interviewing them would be the method of administering the questionnaire. Despite the time-consuming effort and the cost of long-distance calling, all the data would be collected.

From previous experience with administering phone questionnaires, I knew this would be an extremely time-consuming approach because the patient may have other problems that he needs resolved prior to completing the questionnaire. Considering that frequent completion of the questionnaires would be necessary until the patient was "dry," however, we decided that phoning was the approach that would least burden the patient.

Qualitative Versus Quantitative Data

The objective measure of when the radical prostatectomy patients regained urinary continence was the primary goal of this project; an important secondary goal, however, was to learn about the experience of incontinence from the patient's perspective. Because there is a dearth of literature on this topic, we added open-ended questions at the start of the interview to probe how patients perceived and managed their incontinence. Following these questions, the majority of the questionnaire included quantitative items measuring physiologic functioning. Physiologic measures, as defined by Waltz, Strickland, and Lenz (1991), seek to quantify the level of functioning of living beings. The objective of this project was to quantify the level of urinary functioning of these patients following their surgeries—specifically the length of time to continence.

Norm Referenced or Criterion Referenced

The next decision involved the question of whether this would be a norm-referenced or criterion-referenced measure. This is a crucial step for guiding the design and interpretation of any measurement activity. Norm-referenced measures are employed when the interest is in evaluating the performance of a subject relative to the performance of other subjects in some well-defined comparison or norm group (Waltz et al., 1991). In contrast, the sole purpose of a criterion-referenced measure is to determine whether or not a subject has acquired a predetermined set of target behaviors (Waltz et al., 1991). Because we were interested in describing how much the time to regaining continence varied and how the patterns of recovery varied among the patients, a norm-referenced measure was employed. This would provide us with data such as "At Postoperative Week 5, 10% of the patients were wearing three or more liner-type pads during a 24-hour period, 70% were wearing two liner-type pads during a 24-hour period, 12% were wearing one liner-type pad during a 24-hour period, and 8% were totally dry."

Essential steps in the design of a norm-referenced measure are (a) the selection of a conceptual model for delineating the nursing aspects of the measurement process; (b) explication of objectives for the measure; (c) development of a blueprint; and (d) construction of the measure, including administration procedures, an item set, and scoring rules and procedures (Waltz et al., 1991, p. 109).

Harry Herr's Quality of Life and Incontinent Men After Radical Prostatectomy instrument was selected to serve as a conceptual model to aid in clarifying and specifying the purpose of the measurement of urinary incontinence. It provided the structure that was appropriate for the questionnaire. This process led to the explication of the following objectives:

> Primary objective: To determine when patients undergoing a radical prostatectomy regain their urinary continence
>
> Secondary objectives:
>
>> To describe when patients experience any periods or time frames of urinary continence
>>
>> To quantify the level of urinary incontinence being experienced by this population
>>
>> To describe the quality of the patient's urinary stream

Together, the urologist and I first developed a blueprint to emphasize the scope of the questionnaire that eventually evolved into specific questions. For example, to determine when the patient is going to regain urinary continence, it is important to realize that urinary control generally returns in three phases (Walsh & Worthington, 1995). During Phase 1, the patient is dry while in the supine position. In Phase 2, the patient is dry while walking around, and in Phase 3 the patient is dry when standing up after sitting.

We next decided on the best arrangement of the questions to ensure an easy flow of information from the patient during the phone interview. The instrument we developed has three sections and addresses each of the secondary objectives. The first section reviews continence and contains three questions. The second section covers information on the use of pads and contains six questions. The final section addresses the quality of the patient's urinary stream and contains three questions.

MEASURING THE PATIENT OUTCOME

A total of 51 patients were entered into the study. These patients were acquired during a 3-month period, and data collection lasted 6 months for each patient following surgery. Therefore, the data collection period lasted 9 months. Each patient was called and interviewed 2 weeks after his urinary catheter was removed, which was 3 weeks following surgery. The patient was then called and interviewed every 2 weeks until he was dry or until 3 months following surgery and then every month thereafter. During each phone interview, I asked the same questions in the same manner, beginning with "Tell me about your dryness." This was consistent throughout all of the interviews. I found that this approach provided a wealth of information and allowed the patient to talk for awhile before I started asking several questions.

On a personal note, I was amazed at how readily these gentlemen described their experiences with incontinence, how appreciative they were of my calls, and how much they reported looking forward to hearing from someone on a regular basis. This has opened a new area of interest for me to explore—the idea of "coaching." During the development of the questionnaire, the urologist and I decided that the only encouragement that would be shared with the patients during their interviews was to reiterate the need for them to interrupt their urinary stream once during each void to improve their continence. I am curious as to how much impact this encouragement had on the outcomes for this group because they heard this encouragement on a repeated basis, whereas other patients only heard it once as they were discharged from the hospital.

ANALYZING THE DATA

Descriptive statistics were primarily used to analyze the data from this project. Demographic variables such as age were described using the mean and standard deviation. Frequency data were used to describe variables such as the number of patients wearing one or less pads during a 24-hour period or the percentage of patients who had achieved dryness at the selected interview periods.

SUMMARIZING THE FINDINGS

The following was the most important question providing data for the project's primary objective: "What was the date that you last wore a pad?" The number of weeks between the answer to this question and the surgical date were calculated for each of the patients who reached the dry state by the end of 6 months. Of the 51 patients, 34 (66.7%) were experiencing urinary continence 6 months postsurgery. Of the remaining 17 patients, 14 (27.4%) were wearing one or less pads every 24 hours—meaning they were wearing the pad "just in case." For example, many men wear a pad to the gym or when they expect to be engaging in an activity that involves a level of physical stress that may cause them to leak urine. This is considered mild incontinence. Only 3 men (5.9%) were experiencing moderate incontinence or requiring more than one pad every 24 hours. These

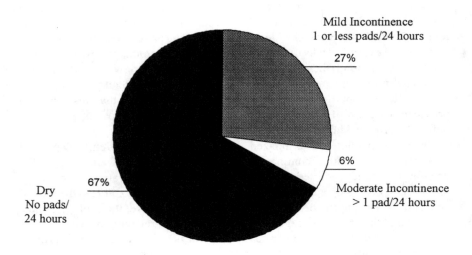

Figure 13.1. Level of Urinary Continence 6 Months Post Radical Prostatectomy
($N = 51$)

were men who have regained urinary continence in the supine and standing positions but still experience some leakage of urine when standing after being in the sitting position. None of the 51 patients in this sample experienced total incontinence (Figure 13.1).

Of the 34 patients who eventually regained their continence, 18 (53%) had regained their continence by Week 7. Interestingly, Week 7 is usually when men are returning to work following their surgery.

Another interesting finding was that all the patients in their 40s had regained their continence by Week 7. The impact that age will have on return of urinary continence is a major concern for many men. Table 13.1 was created to summarize the average age and age range of patients according to the week that the regaining of urinary continence was achieved.

For the 34 patients who did achieve continence, Figure 13.2 depicts the number of patients regaining urinary continence by each postoperative week. For example, on Postoperative Week 4, three men regained their urinary continence.

Overall, the findings of this project are limited by several factors. First, because the instrument is new, additional studies must be undertaken to further test its reliability. Another limitation is that a sample size of 51 is not large enough to generalize study findings to the population of patients undergoing radical prostatectomy. Using only the patients of one urologist further limits the

TABLE 13.1 Urinary Continence Summary With Average Age and Age Range
$(N = 51)$

Week Postsurgery	% Dry	Average Age	Age Range
3	2	63	63
4	6	61.3	56-67
5	12	57.3	47-61
6	6	52.3	46-59
7	10	61.8	48-68
8	4	53.5	53-54
9	6	63.3	61-65
10	4	58.5	56-61
11	2	66	66
12	2	60	60
13	4	64	60-68
17	2	62	62
26	8	56.8	54-62

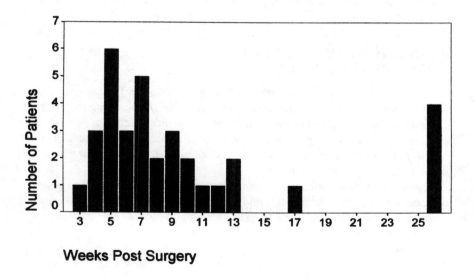

Figure 13.2. Number of Weeks Post Radical Prostatectomy Patients Experienced No Urinary Incontinence $(N = 34)$

generalizability of findings. Despite these limitations, this exploratory study contributed to our knowledge development in several ways: (a) It alerted the urological group to include this measurement in two additional studies; (b) it helped to identify other areas that are in need of study, such as why some men remain dry all day but still leak urine at night; and (c) it led to the refinement of the questionnaire to include the addition of pad weighing.

APPLYING THE FINDINGS
TO PRACTICE

The primary objective of this project was to provide data regarding when patients undergoing a radical prostatectomy regain their urinary continence so that the data could be shared with patients preparing to have the procedure. We consider the results of this initial study too preliminary to share with patients, but we are working toward this goal as we continue our study of incontinence. One important outcome of the study has been a heightened awareness on our part of the need to spend more time talking with patients about incontinence. I now tell patients,

> The staff at this institution realizes that regaining your urinary continence is a major concern for you. We are here to help you with this and continue to study this important problem so that we may understand how to best help patients recover following surgery.

PLANNING FUTURE PATIENT
OUTCOMES PROJECTS

As mentioned previously, this questionnaire is being used in two additional studies. One study is reviewing the impact that a new surgical approach to radical prostatectomy (known as the minilap) has on urinary incontinence. Another project is studying the impact that urinary incontinence has on the quality of life of the radical prostatectomy patient. This project will review more than 200 patients from eight urologists.

Other factors associated with urinary incontinence that need further research include age, weight, and alcohol and caffeine intake. Each of these factors is thought to possibly contribute to urinary incontinence in the prostatectomy patient.

REFERENCES

Fowler, F., Wennberg, J., Timothy, R., Barry, M., Mulley, A., & Hanley, D. (1988). Symptom status and quality of life following prostatectomy. *Journal of the American Medical Association, 259*(20), 3018-3022.

Gittes, R. (1991). Carcinoma of the prostate. *New England Journal of Medicine, 324,* 236-245.

Herr, H. (1994). Quality of life of incontinent men after radical prostatectomy. *Journal of Urology, 151,* 652-654.

Walsh, P., & Worthington, J. (1995). *The prostate: A guide for men and the women who love them.* Baltimore, MD: Johns Hopkins University Press.

Waltz, C., Strickland, O., & Lenz, E. (1991). *Measurement in nursing research* (2nd ed.). Philadelphia: Davis.

POSTPROSTATECTOMY CONTINENCE
SERIAL FOLLOW-UP

Name: _____DOB _____

Medical Record Number: _____DOS _____

Date of Phoning: _____/_____/_____   Week # _____

CONTINENCE:

1. How much dryness do you experience?

2. In what positions are you dry?

	Supine	Y	N
	Sitting	Y	N
	Standing	Y	N

3. How much effort is required to produce leakage?
   Activity level _____

PADS:

1. How many pads do you use in 24 hours? _____

2. What brand _____ and size _____ of pad are you using?

3. How frequently are you changing the pad? _____

4. How wet are the pads you discard?

Damp	Y	N
Wet	Y	N
Soaked	Y	N

5. Do you wear a pad at night?   Y   N

6. What was the date that you last wore a pad?   _____/_____/_____

STREAM:

1. Is it good?   Y   N

2. Is it continuous or intermittent?

3. Does it project away from your body or dribble?

NOTE: At 2 or 3 months postop, interrupt stream once during each void to improve continence.

CHAPTER 14

A Clinical Outcomes Study to Evaluate the Cost-Effectiveness of New Antiemetic Guidelines for the Management of Chemotherapy-Related Nausea and Vomiting

Christine A. Engstrom

EDITORS' NOTE: Sometimes, symptom management is the most important outcome to patients. This chapter describes the use of an oral antiemetic guideline to manage nausea in cancer patients receiving chemotherapy. Using patient-recorded diaries, the author was able to obtain an accurate evaluation of this outcome. The guideline proved to be a safe and effective way to manage nausea in this cancer population and achieved a cost savings when compared to the former intravenous antiemetic regimen.

IDENTIFYING THE PATIENT OUTCOME

A major goal in the treatment and supportive care of cancer patients is the control of chemotherapy-induced emesis. The severity of emesis has been greatly reduced in most patients whose symptoms were refractory to the older antiemetic regimens, and in many cases the emesis is now prevented (Gralla, 1997). It is well documented that the incidence and severity of nausea and vomiting in patients receiving chemotherapy depend on the emetic potential of the chemotherapeutic agent, its dose and schedule of administration, and individual patient variables (Cubeddu, 1992). The recent use of the 5-HT3 (serotonin) antagonists combined with corticosteroids represents a significant advance in the supportive care of these patients (Cleri, 1996; Ettinger, 1995; Perez, 1995). The combination of the 5-HT3 antagonists and corticosteroids such as dexamethasone has replaced previously used varying combinations of metroclopramide, prochlorperazine, and dexamethasone in the treatment of acute nausea and vomiting induced by chemotherapy. Recent studies have demonstrated that oral formulations of both ondansetron and granisetron are as safe, effective, and perhaps less expensive than the intravenous preparations for acute nausea and vomiting (Beck, 1992; Hainsworth & Hasketh, 1992; Perez, 1995). These agents have become the antiemetics of choice because they provide major protection from nausea and vomiting in 70% to 90% of patients receiving high or moderately high emetogenic chemotherapy (Ettinger et al., 1996).

Despite positive reports of the effectiveness of these oral antiemetics, several questions remain regarding the most appropriate use of these drugs. The optimal dose, the route and frequency of administration, and their usefulness in managing delayed nausea and vomiting are controversial. The 5-HT3 antagonists do not appear to be superior to metoclopramide or prochlorperazine for delayed nausea and vomiting after high-dose cisplatin when used in combination with a corticosteriod (Gralla, 1997).

The rapid acceptance of the 5-HT3 antagonists in the 1990s into clinical practice has been accompanied by some misuse of these agents. Prior to the introduction of antiemetic guidelines at our institution, most patients received 32 mg of ondansetron intravenously (i.v.) for the prevention of acute nausea and vomiting, regardless of the emetogenic potential of the chemotherapeutic regimen. There was no consistent regimen for the control of delayed emesis, and patients were frequently admitted to the hospital with dehydration and uncontrolled nausea and vomiting following chemotherapy administration.

As the oncology nurse practitioner, I worked with the clinical nurse specialist, the clinical pharmacist, and the oncologist to develop antiemetic guidelines that would increase patient compliance with the antiemetic regimens, improve the effectiveness of the antiemetics used, optimize nursing and pharmacy time, and enhance cost savings for the institution.

BUILDING THE TEAM

We held organized interdisciplinary staff meetings every other week in the outpatient oncology department of our institution to discuss issues regarding the oncology inpatients and outpatients. Our outpatient staff consisted of a clinical oncologist, an oncology nurse practitioner, an oncology clinical nurse specialist, a dietician, a social worker, and a clinical pharmacist. We had developed an interdisciplinary clinical pathway and performance improvement plan for chemotherapy-induced nausea and vomiting. Oral 5-HT3 antagonists were beginning to be used in chemotherapy-induced emesis at that time. Although we had limited experience using the oral regimens, pharmaceutical companies had forwarded convincing evidence from clinical trials that had been performed in the United States and Europe.

The clinical oncologist was interested in evaluating an all-oral antiemetic regimen, and this idea was presented to us at one of our staff meetings. We decided this would be a project that could lead to increased comfort for patients and cost savings in care delivery. At that time, our patients were receiving their antiemetics as i.v. infusions prior to the administration of chemotherapy, which took 30 to 45 minutes depending on the regimen ordered. The time for preparation and administration of the medications was also a consideration. Many patients had been hospitalized due to intractable nausea and vomiting and dehydration following chemotherapy administration. We are affiliated with a large teaching institution and have several oncology fellows and attending physicians who rotate through our oncology department. Because there were no antiemetic guidelines to follow, there was little consistency in the antiemetic regimens ordered for both acute and delayed nausea and vomiting.

Our project began with a literature search of research on oral antiemetics. It was at this time that our dietician and social worker decided that they would not participate in the project but would be available for consultation if needed. I conducted the literature search and reviewed articles relevant to the project. The clinical nurse specialist contacted the two pharmaceutical companies that produced the 5-HT3 receptors to enlist their aid in obtaining research articles relevant to the project. Both of the companies were very receptive and cooperative, providing abstracts, articles, and information on clinical trials in progress. After briefly reviewing the articles, we selected those that were relevant to bring to our next meeting, during which we divided them among the group for critique.

Group members reviewed several articles and presented their critiques at the next meeting. Because we found no published guidelines regarding an all-oral antiemetic regimen for chemotherapy-induced nausea and vomiting, we were confident that our study would be valuable to both patients and clinicians.

We agreed to conduct a clinical outcomes study that would describe the effectiveness of an all-oral antiemetic regimen to manage chemotherapy-induced nausea. In addition, the cost of the proposed oral regimen would be compared with the cost of the traditional i.v. antiemetic regimen used prior to this study. A final objective was to develop standard clinical guidelines for antiemetics. The following sections provide a summary of the role that each team member played in the project.

Oncology Clinical Nurse Specialist and Nurse Practitioner

We reviewed the research articles and clinical trials that had been conducted on oral antiemetics. We used this information to develop instruments to measure patient satisfaction and compliance as well as a method of tracking the number of emetic episodes. The tools needed to be brief, clear, and easy for the patients and for us to use to collect the data. These tasks took several weeks to complete because we were doing this study in addition to our other daily responsibilities. We explained the study to the patients and taught them how to complete the patient diary. The two of us were responsible for all the data collection and interpretation as well as for initiating the write-up of the study (Engstrom, Hernandez, Haywood, & Lilenbaum, 1999).

Clinical Oncologist

The oncologist's role was to develop the antiemetic guidelines. He did this by reviewing journal articles and abstracts to develop the most effective oral regimen for the patients. He also defined the eligibility and ineligibility criteria for the patients who would be candidates for an all-oral regimen. In addition, he served as coauthor for the publication describing this study.

Clinical Pharmacist

The pharmacist reviewed the medical records of all patients who had received chemotherapy during the 9 months prior to this project to determine the frequency of use of i.v. and oral antiemetics. She compared this use with the use of oral antiemetics during the 9 months following the introduction of the all-oral antiemetic regimen. The pharmacist calculated the cost of nursing and pharmacy time for the provision of each regimen based on the time it takes to prepare and administer the drugs. The cost of the drugs and the supplies used in their preparation and administration was also included in the analysis. Finally, the pharmacist participated in the publication of the project.

SELECTING THE INSTRUMENTS

Once we had collected data on previous antiemetic practices and costs and reviewed the literature, we met again to present our work to the group. I had collected instruments that had been used in previous clinical trials to evaluate nausea and vomiting.

Patient Diary

The patient diary was 1 page in length and designed to be easy for patients to increase patient compliance in completing the form. The diary was developed to measure the effectiveness of and patient satisfaction with the new oral antiemetic regimen. Patients were asked to complete the diary each evening at bedtime for 7 days following chemotherapy administration. They recorded the number of emetic episodes from Day 1 through Day 7. Satisfaction with the control of nausea and vomiting was measured using a 100-mm visual analog scale.

The primary measure of vomiting was the number of emetic episodes recorded by the patient and ratings of how it interfered with daily life. An emetic episode was defined as a single occurrence of retching, vomiting, or any number of continuous occurrences of retching and vomiting followed by the absence of both nausea and vomiting for at least 1 minute. The number of emetic episodes experienced by the patient defined the response to treatment during each 24-hour period. Mild nausea without vomiting was defined as a complete response, one or two emetic episodes were a major response, three to five episodes were a minor response, and more than five episodes were considered a failure of the regimen.

The patients were asked to indicate the severity of nausea each day with a check mark next to descriptions that were rated as follows: 0, no nausea; 1, mild but did not interfere with activities of daily living; 2, moderately interfered with activities of daily living; or 3, severe and bedridden due to nausea. They were also asked to record the dates and times the antiemetics were taken and any additional medications taken for nausea. The diary ended with the statement, "Did you experience any side effects related to your antinausea medication and if so please list them." The patients were asked to return the diary to the nurses the following week at the clinic. Patients receiving chemotherapy have blood samples collected on a weekly basis in our hospital lab, thus providing us with the opportunity to encourage compliance with the completion of the diaries.

Nursing Data Collection Tool

The nurses devised a 2-page tool to collect demographic and treatment information on the patients, including the chemotherapy data. The first page listed the drug information, including the dates, agents, doses, and times they were given. The second page was used to record the responses to treatment from the patient diaries. It was from this page that we extracted the data for analyses.

Standard Antiemetic Order Form

The oncologist and pharmacist designed a 1-page order sheet. The front of the form listed the four regimens: one for patients receiving highly or moderately high emetogenic agents, one for those receiving moderately emetogenic agents, one for those receiving mildly emetogenic agents, and one for delayed nausea and vomiting. The clinician checked the desired regimen and signed the order sheet to complete it. The reverse side of the order form contained the emetogenic classification of the chemotherapeutic agents and commonly used combinations of agents.

MEASURING THE PATIENT OUTCOME

A total of 52 patients seen in the outpatient oncology clinic served as the sample for this project. For a 9-month period, patients received the oral antiemetic regimen. Patients normally returned to the clinic on a weekly basis for blood testing. During these visits, they were encouraged to complete their antiemetic diary. When we encountered patients who forgot to bring their diaries to the clinic, we encouraged them to bring them the following week. We knew that some patients would have difficulty remembering to complete the diaries, and for these patients we enlisted the aid of their support person(s). We also would call the patient's home the night before the clinic visit to improve compliance. We found ourselves hand-writing the instructions for the delayed emesis regimen for every patient and verbally giving the information. Toward the end of the study, we computerized a calendar for the patients. Thus, it was very simple for us to write in the dates of the medications and give a copy of the calendar to the patients and families.

The antiemetic order sheet and a cover memorandum were sent to all the oncology attending physicians and fellows at the initiation of the study. A few of the attending physicians voiced concern regarding the guidelines, stating that they did not want medical practice dictated to them. This became less of an issue when it was explained to them that these were "guidelines" to practice. It has become standard practice to use the antiemetic order form and the oral regimen for most patients, however. The cost of oral antiemetic therapy was evaluated by comparing it to the cost of i.v. antiemetic therapy that was provided in the same oncology clinic during the 9-month period prior to this study.

ANALYZING THE DATA

Fifty-two patients were enrolled in the study between September 1995 and May 1996. The pharmacist devised a spreadsheet using Excel (1996) to manage all our data. The descriptive statistics are summarized in Table 14.1. The extent to

TABLE 14.1 Characteristics of Patients Receiving the All-Oral Antiemetic Regimen ($N = 52$)

Characteristic	n
Sex	
Female	1
Male	51
Age, years	
Median	64
Range	39-76
Outpatient	41
Inpatient	11
Cancer diagnosis	
Lung	24
Head/neck	6
Colon	5
Esophageal	4
Unknown primary	3
Lymphoma	3
Bladder	2
Prostate/breast	1/1
Gastric/pancreatic	1/1
Chronic lymphocytic lymphoma	1

which patients responded to the oral antiemetic regimen by the emetogenic potential of the chemotherapy they received is summarized in Table 14.2. Results of the comparison of the cost of the oral antiemetic regimen described in this study with that of i.v. antiemetic regimen used prior to this study are summarized in Figure 14.1.

SUMMARIZING THE FINDINGS

Patient compliance was excellent (100%) with recording the antiemetic medications every day. No PRN medications were taken by any of the patients, and no toxicities were reported. Also, the mean score on the 100-mm visual analog scale for patient satisfaction was 89 mm, indicating high overall satisfaction with the control of nausea and vomiting.

TABLE 14.2 Patient Responses to an All-Oral Antiemetic Regimen During the First
24 Hours by Chemotherapy Emetogenic Potential

Chemotherapy Emetogenic Potential (n)	Response % (n)			
	Complete	Major	Minor	Failure
High (29)	79.3 (23)	13.8 (4)	0	6.9 (2)
Moderate (6)	100 (6)	0	0	0
Mild (17)	100 (17)	0	0	0

Patient responses during the first 24 hours after chemotherapy by the chemo-therapy emetogenic potential are summarized in Table 14.2. For the patients who received the delayed regimen from Days 2 to 7, complete protection was demonstrated in 50% of the patients and a major response in 21% of them. No episodes of extrapyramidal reactions were reported despite the relatively high doses of prochlorperazine. We were also pleased that there were no toxicities experienced with the serotonin antagonists because the literature reports an approximate 20% incidence of headache with the medication (Ettinger et al., 1996). In addition, the study findings confirmed previously published observa-tions that serotonin antagonists are not necessary for delayed nausea and vomit-ing. The combination of prochlorperazine and dexamethasone has proven to be safe and effective in delayed emesis.

Our results demonstrated that the all-oral antiemetic regimens included in our guidelines were both safe and effective when targeted to the emetic potential of each chemotherapeutic drug or combination of drugs. The effectiveness of all-oral combinations appears to be comparable to the effectiveness of intrave-nous preparations that have been described in the literature. Intravenous antiemetics are more costly, take more time to prepare and administer, and are not ideal in the home or ambulatory setting. The time saved by eliminating the need for administration of intravenous antiemetics can be quite substantial in a busy treatment center (Rhodes, McDaniel, Simms, & Johnson, 1995).

APPLYING THE FINDINGS TO PRACTICE

The results of this study have had a dramatic effect on clinical practice in our institution. We have adhered to the clinical guidelines of the project and rarely use intravenous preparations. The few patients who have dysphagia or odynophagia continue to receive the i.v. preparations.

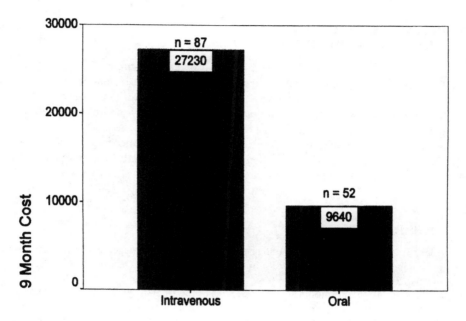

Figure 14.1. Antiemetic Cost Comparison: Intravenous Versus Oral Regimen (Total Savings of Oral Regimen, $17,591)

We have demonstrated the guidelines to be cost-effective. The oral antiemetic regimens used for 9 months in this study resulted in actual cost savings of $17,591.22 when compared with the cost of i.v. regimens used in the 9 months prior to this study. These results have been presented at interdisciplinary staff meetings within the institution with rave reviews.

The dramatic increase in health care cost, coupled with decreased financial resources, has stimulated a focus on the cost-effectiveness of nursing and medical treatment. We were able to make a positive financial impact on our institution with our project. The amount of cost savings surprised all of us. Prior to the study, we had not fully considered the cost of medications or the monetary value of our nursing time. We have educated the staff members in the inpatient nursing units about the oral antiemetic guidelines and the procedures that make it easier for them to administer the medications.

The project took only 9 months to complete because we used a convenience sample of patients in our outpatient department. Conducting research that led to the improvement of clinical practice was a challenging experience for all of us who participated. The most rewarding part of the experience has been observing the patients' improved clinical response to these practice changes.

PLANNING FUTURE PATIENT OUTCOMES PROJECTS

We plan to improve on this patient outcome project in the future. Our guidelines for mildly emetogenic chemotherapy use a serotonin antagonist prior to treatment. The patients who refused to participate in our project did so because they had previously received a mildly emetogenic medication and did not believe they needed antiemetics. We wish to repeat a portion of the study using these particular patients who received mildly emetogenic chemotherapy, collecting the same data on efficacy and patient satisfaction using PRN antiemetics. Outcome measures would be satisfaction, efficacy, and cost-effectiveness.

REFERENCES

Beck, T. M. (1992). Efficacy of ondansetron tablets in the management of chemotherapy induced emesis: Review of clinical trials. *Seminars in Oncology, 19* (6, Suppl. 15), 20-25.

Cleri, R. B. (1996). Serotonin antagonists: State of the art management of chemotherapy induced emesis. *Oncology Nursing Treatment and Support, 2,* 1-19.

Cubeddu, L. X. (1992). Mechanisms by which cancer chemotherapeutic drugs induce emesis. *Seminars in Oncology, 19*(6, Suppl. 15), 2-13.

Engstrom, C., Hernandez, I., Haywood, J., & Lilenbaum, R. (1999). The efficacy and cost effectiveness of new anti-emetic guidelines. *Oncology Nursing Forum, 26*(9), 1453-1458.

Ettinger, D. (1995). Preventing chemotherapy induced nausea and vomiting. An update and review of emesis. *Seminars in Oncology, 22*(4, Suppl. 10), 6-18.

Ettinger, D., Eisenberg, P., Fitts, D., Friedman, C., Wilson-Lynch, K., & Yocum, K. (1996). A double blind comparison of the efficacy of two dose regimens of oral granisetron, in preventing acute emesis in patients receiving moderately emetogenic chemotherapy. *American Cancer Society, 78,* 144-151.

Excel 97 for Windows [Computer software]. (1996). Redmond, WA: Microsoft.

Gralla, R. (1997). Anti-emesis with cancer chemotherapy. *European Journal of Cancer, 33*(Suppl. 4), 63-67.

Hainsworth, J., & Hasketh, P. (1992). Single dose ondansetron for prevention of cisplatin induced emesis: Efficacy results. *Seminars in Oncology, 10*(6, Suppl. 15), 14-19.

Perez, E. (1995). Oral granisetron (Kytril tablets): Prophylaxis for chemotherapy induced nausea and vomiting. *Seminars in Oncology, 22*(4, Suppl. 10), 1-2.

Rhodes, V., McDaniel, R. W., Simms, S. G., & Johnson, M. (1995). Nurse's perception of anti-emetic effectiveness. *Oncology Nursing Forum, 11*(8), 1243-1252.

Glossary

Agency for Health Care Policy and Research—a federal agency that supports and disseminates research dealing with patient outcomes; provides online data on the Internet on length of stay and mean charges by diagnostic-related groups.

ANOVA/ANCOVA (analysis of variance/analysis of covariance)—a statistical procedure to determine differences among two or more group means. In ANCOVA, the subjects are made statistically equal on a potentially confounding variable (the covariable).

Benchmark—to compare the care processes and outcomes of one group of patients with those of a similar group of patients in another organization known for having the best practice in this type of care. This method can be used to identify an organization's areas of weakness and to prioritize the patient outcomes on which to focus.

Boxplot—a summary plot based on the median, quartiles, and extreme values. The box represents the interquartile range that contains the 50% of values. The whiskers are lines that extend from the box to the highest and lowest values, excluding outliers. A line across the box indicates the median.

Capitation—a method of reimbursement for health care services that includes a flat fee per subscriber regardless of the amount of health services provided.

Case manager—a person who oversees the care of groups of patients through collaboration with other health professionals, coordination of services, and elimination of inefficiencies in the delivery of care.

Chi-square (χ^2)—a statistical test used to determine if there is a difference between frequencies of two categorical variables, such as the difference between groups on gender, education, types of employment, or religion.

Contingency table—a cross-tabulation table exhibiting the frequencies of two variables within a sample.

Copyright—the legal right to publish, reproduce, or market a creative work, such as a computer program or an artistic or literary composition.

Correlation—describes the strength of the relationship between two variables.

Correlation coefficient—numerical account of the relationship between two variables; values can range from −1 to 1, where 0 = no relationship, 1 = the strongest positive relationship (A + B increase together), and −1 = strongest negative or inverse relationship (as A increases, B decreases).

Critical pathway—a written schedule of treatments and interventions for patients within the same diagnostic group or who are undergoing a similar procedure. The objective of the pathway is to decrease fragmentation of services and cost of care.

Cronbach's alpha—a reliability index that assesses the extent to which items in an instrument, such as questions on a survey, are related. On a scale of 0 to 1.0, higher values reflect a higher degree of internal consistency.

Descriptive statistics—statistics used to describe and summarize data (e.g., frequency, mean, and percentages).

Diagnostic-related group—a system of categorizing patients for the purpose of reimbursement according to factors such as diagnosis, procedure, and comorbidities; first developed within the Medicare program.

Effectiveness of care—the extent to which interventions achieve the desired outcomes when applied in the practice setting.

Efficacy of care—the extent to which interventions achieve the desired outcome in a controlled setting.

External validity—the generalizability of the study's results to other samples or settings.

Fee-for-services—a method of reimbursement for health care services in which payment is provided for the health care services delivered.

Frequency distribution—a display of numerical values from lowest to highest with a count of the number of times each value was observed.

Health maintenance organization (HMO)—a health care organization that uses primary physicians to control subscriber access to care within designated health care facilities; the objective is to decrease costs by limiting the care provided.

Heterogeneity—the degree to which objects are dissimilar or varied with respect to some attribute.

Histogram—displays the distribution of a quantitative variable by showing the relative concentration of data points along different intervals or sections of the scale on which the data are measured.

Homogeneity—the degree to which objects are similar or equivalent with respect to some attribute.

Hypothesis—a statement predicting the relationship between two or more variables.

Inferential statistics—used for making generalizations from samples to populations and in estimating or testing population parameters or hypotheses using samples of the population.

Instruments, tools, and measures—the methods or devices used to collect data (e.g., questionnaire).

Internal validity—the extent to which it can be inferred that the independent variable in a study, rather than extraneous factors, is responsible for the outcomes (dependent variables).

Interrater reliability—the extent that two independent raters assign the same value for a characteristic (a specific variable) being measured.

Interval—level of measurement in which an attribute of a variable is rank ordered with equal numerical distances between points on a scale (e.g., temperature).

Kruskall-Wallis test—a nonparametric statistical test used to detect differences among three or more independent groups when the data are an ordinal level of measurement.

Level of significance (or alpha)—the risk of rejecting a null hypothesis when it is true (Type I error). The cutoff point resolves whether the sample tested is of the same or a different population.

Mann-Whitney *U* test—a nonparametric statistical test used to detect differences between two independent groups based on ordinal data.

Mean—the arithmetic average score computed by adding all scores and dividing by the number of scores.

Median—the middle score in a set of numbers; half of the set is higher than and half is lower than the middle score.

Mode—most frequently occurring score in a data set.

National Committee for Quality Assurance—the private, not-for-profit organization that accredits managed care organizations. This organization examines several key indicators of quality of care, such as patient satisfaction and frequency of childhood immunization.

Nominal—lowest level of measurement. Variables with similar characteristics are assigned a label. If a number label is used, it is arbitrary (not used for arithmetic purposes).

Nonparametric test—statistical test used with a sample when the rigorous assumptions about a normal distribution of scores on a variable are not met; generally used with data measured on nominal and ordinal scales.

Normal distribution—a continuous frequency distribution of scores that is bell-shaped, symmetrical, and unimodal.

Null hypothesis—states that there is no relationship between the variables being studied; a form of the hypothesis used for statistical testing.

Ordinal—level of measurement that involves rank ordering of data where the intervals (differences in order of magnitude between ranks) are not equal.

Outcome—the end result of care or a measurable change in the health status or behavior of patients. Outcomes may be clinical, functional, financial, or perceptual.

Outlier—extreme numerical score that lies remotely from the center of a distribution of scores.

p **Value or alpha level**—the level of probability that the obtained results are a result of chance (probability of a Type I error). Generally, .05 alpha level means that generalizing to the real world or in repeating the study one should find these same differences 95 out of 100 times; thus, it is unlikely that the differences are due to chance.

Parametric test—a statistical test used when the assumption of normal distribution of scores or values can be met and the level of measurement is interval or ratio; considered more powerful than nonparametric tests (e.g., *t* test).

Pearson's *r* (Pearson's product-moment correlation coefficient)—a parametric statistical test used to determine magnitude and direction of the relationship between variables.

Population (target)—the total set of objects that have some common attribute and meet the specific criteria for a research study.

Power—the probability that a statistical test will detect a significant relationship among variables if one exists.

Preferred provider organization—a health care network involving contracts with groups of physicians and other health professionals to provide care for a reduced rate in return for an increased volume of patients; less restrictive than an HMO because no gatekeeper physician is used to limit access to care.

Range—a measure of variability obtained by subtracting the lowest from the highest score in a distribution of scores.

Ratio—highest level of measurement. There are equal numerical distances between points on the scale and a true meaningful zero point (e.g., heart rate).

Reliability—the consistency or repeatability with which an instrument measures the attribute it is designed to measure.

Sample—the portion of the population that is selected to participate in a research study.

Scatterplot—a graph in which one numeric variable is plotted against another.

Selectivity—the ability of an instrument to correctly identify the presence of an attribute being measured and to distinguish it from similar attributes.

Sensitivity—the ability of an instrument to detect differing amounts of the attribute being measured.

Spearman's rho (Spearman's rank-order correlation coefficient)—a nonparametric statistical test used to determine relationships between two variables measured at the ordinal level.

Standard deviation (square root of the variance)—the average deviation of scores from the mean of all scores in the data set.

Statistical significance—the extent to which the results are not due to chance at some specific level of probability.

Subjects—individuals participating in a research study.

t **test**—parametric statistical test used for analyzing differences between the mean scores of two groups.

Type I error—error that occurs when the null hypothesis is rejected when it is actually true (a relationship is concluded to exist when one does not exist).

Type II error—error that occurs when the null hypothesis is accepted when it should have been rejected (a relationship is concluded not to exist when one does exist in reality).

Validity—the degree to which an instrument measures what it is supposed to measure.

Variable—any characteristic or attribute that changes or varies within the population under study.

Variance—The square of the standard deviation. A large variance means that the data are widely distributed.

Index